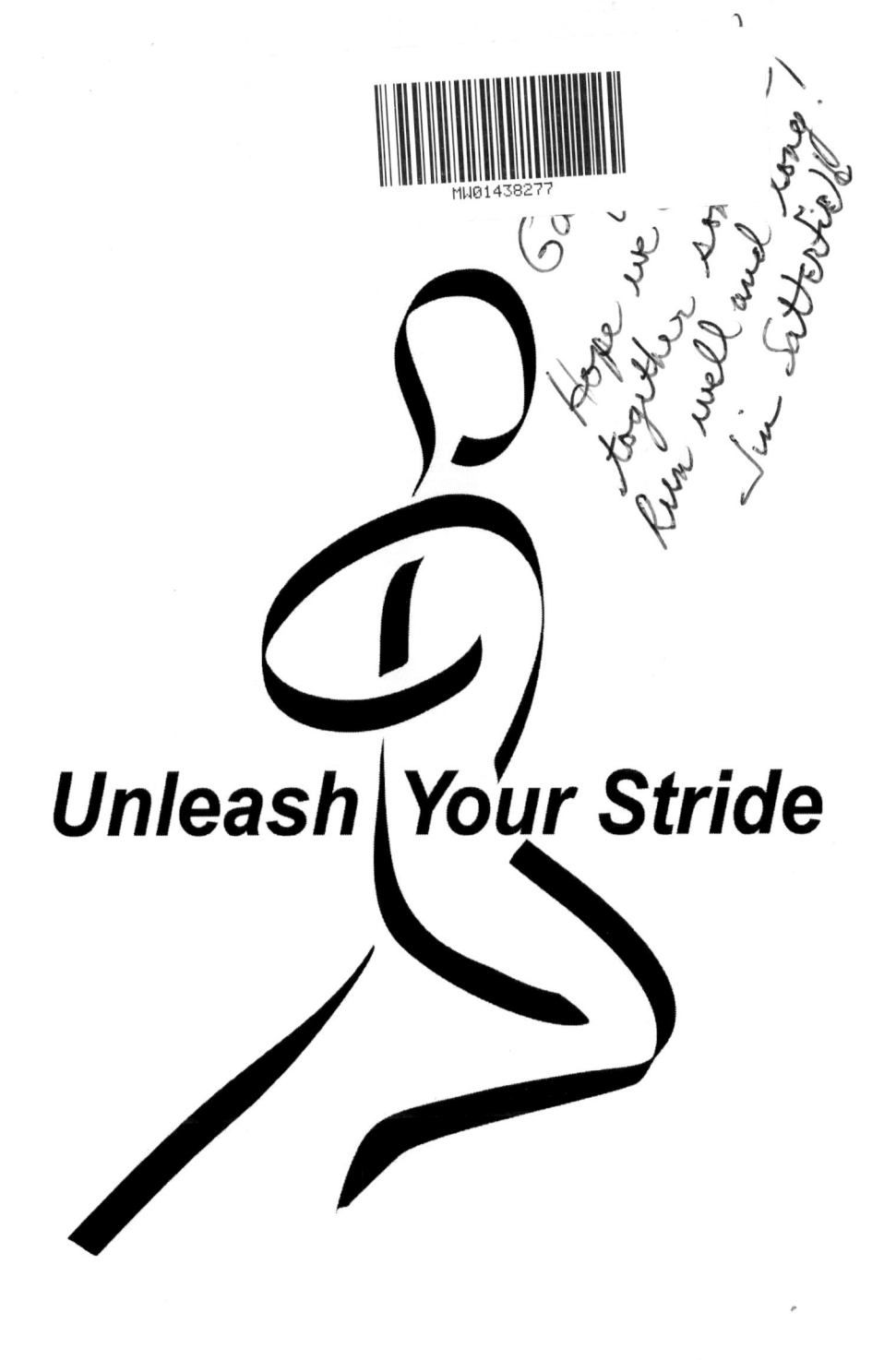

Unleash Your Stride

Unleash Your Stride

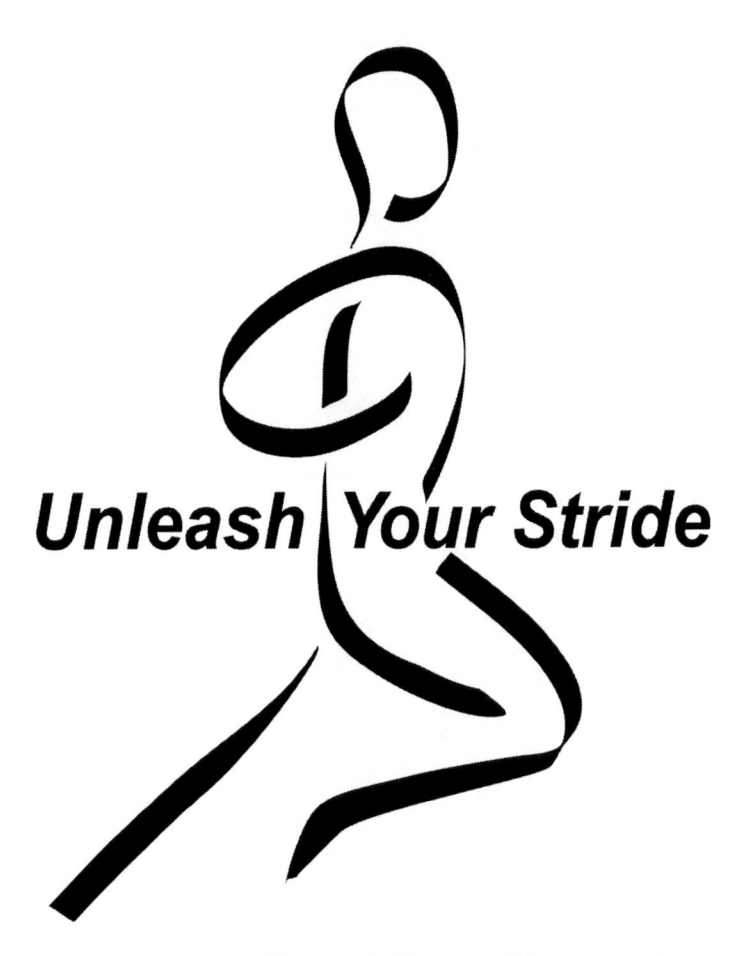

Learn to Run Like a Natural

Jim Satterfield

iUniverse, Inc.
New York Bloomington

Unleash Your Stride

Copyright © 2008, 2010 by Jim Satterfield

All rights reserved. No part of this book may be used or reproduced by any means, graphic, electronic, or mechanical, including photocopying, recording, taping or by any information storage retrieval system without the written permission of the publisher except in the case of brief quotations embodied in critical articles and reviews.

You should not undertake any diet/exercise regimen recommended in this book before consulting your personal physician. Neither the author nor the publisher shall be responsible or liable for any loss or damage allegedly arising as a consequence of your use or application of any information or suggestions contained in this book.

The front and back cover photos, along with the running photos on pages 73, 74 and 75 were taken by "Hall Anderson"

iUniverse books may be ordered through booksellers or by contacting:

iUniverse
1663 Liberty Drive
Bloomington, IN 47403
www.iuniverse.com
1-800-Authors (1-800-288-4677)

Because of the dynamic nature of the Internet, any Web addresses or links contained in this book may have changed since publication and may no longer be valid. The views expressed in this work are solely those of the author and do not necessarily reflect the views of the publisher, and the publisher hereby disclaims any responsibility for them.

ISBN: 978-1-4401-9903-5 (sc)
ISBN: 978-1-4401-9905-9 (dj)
ISBN: 978-1-4401-9904-2 (ebook)

Library of Congress Control Number: 2010921837

Printed in the United States of America

iUniverse rev. date: 04/30/2010

Contents

Acknowledgments vii

Preface ix

1 My Story: From Four-Year-Old Track Star to Coach 1

2 The Coach–Runner Relationship: Sharing the Olympic Dream 19

3 Ready …Warm-up Exercises to Unleash Your Stride 27

    The Pre-Run Routine 33

        Exercise 1: Leading Knee 33

        Exercise 2: Kicking from the Core 35

        Exercise 3: Leading Knee Crunch 39

        Exercise 4: Back Leg Kicks 41

        Exercise 5: Leg Waves 45

        Exercise 6: Push-ups! 47

4 Set … Action Assignments to Run Like a Natural 49

    Drills to Improve Your Stride 61

        Action Assignment 1: Pushing the Wall 61

        Action Assignment 2: Posture Line-up 65

        Action Assignment 3: Stepping in Place 68

        Action Assignment 4: Balancing Your Stride 71

5 Go! Finding the Zone 77

6 Cooling Down—The Importance of Rest and Deciding What's Next 85

Acknowledgments

I'm grateful in so many ways for all that running has done for me. I want to thank those who have helped me along the path of running and also writing this project.

Early on, both my parents recognized and supported my need to be a runner. Pacific Northwest weather can be tough on spectators, but that didn't stop my mom and dad from coming out in the pouring rain to show me how much they cared.

Thanks to my children, Amy and Grant, for the lessons I've learned being their dad and, at times, their coach. I would also like to thank my secretary, Dana Barden, for patiently teaching me how to use my computer and treating me like I was family.

To the people in my life that I have come to know through athletics, thank you. The list includes coaches, competitors, fans, officials, students, and teammates. In one manner or another, they inspired me to write this book, which has allowed me to pass my knowledge of the sport on to others.

To my running mates in the Portland Masters Track Club, Spud Henderson, the Road Dogs, and the East Wind Breakers—thanks for years of friendship and for putting on events that have kept me motivated to train the last twenty-five years.

Thanks to fellow authors Leo Collins, Toni Edey, Marlene Smith-Baranzini, and Mike Rangner for helping me improve my early manuscripts, and the folks at iUniverse for helping with the final product.

Near the completion of this book, I became acquainted with internal martial arts master Harry Affley. We quickly developed a friendship and respect for each other's opinions and devotion to the study of how the human body is designed and should move. Studying with Harry has validated my theories and has deepened my understanding.

Danny Abshire, cofounder and designer of Newton Running Shoes, is also someone I recently met and with whom I share several ideas. He outfitted me for the pictures in the book. To learn more about his revolutionary shoes and to purchase a pair of your own, visit my Web site, www.unleashyourstride.com.

A runner with whom I had been casually acquainted visited my office one day. After we finished talking business, she told me that I needed to meet her cousin. I could see that Janet was going to be persistent, so I agreed to make the call. I'm glad I did, because Leslie and I hit it off right away and soon fell in love. We're now happily married and are blending a new life with both of our families and mutual friends. Even though she's not a runner, Leslie understands and supports my need to run and coach. In fact, she's pushed me like a coach to get this book completed and ready to publish. By marrying Leslie, I also got a new brother-in-law, Hall Anderson, who happens to be a huge fan of track and field and a professional photographer. Thank you, Hall, for taking pictures until we got a few that met with both of our approval.

Preface

This book was written on the premise that all runners should have a fundamentally sound stride, yet few runners seem to find one on their own. Once in a while, you run across a "natural," someone whose stride and ease of running looks like he or she was born to it. They are the exceptions rather than the rule. Most people can run in some manner, but they need to improve their form. After more than fifty years of studying and experimenting, I have developed a method to teach others how to run *like a natural.* Everyone who has been using this method has improved their stride and, consequently, their enjoyment of running.

Mastering the fundamentals is the way to success in *any* activity—including running. What sets this book apart is the way natural running fundamentals are taught through a unique series of lessons. The lessons are designed to teach runners how to begin the movements that are fundamentally correct, and how to discover and eliminate movements that slow runners down. I show how running with better form takes advantage of the way each of us is built and the proven laws of physics. Repeating these lessons and thereby mastering fundamentals will help any runner learn ways to develop and maintain a more natural stride.

I have been a competitive age-group runner since the 1950s. As an athlete and a coach, I have won at the youth, high school, college, open, and master's levels. At one time or another, I have competed in every standard field event in the sport of track and field, and have raced in every standard running and hurdle distance—from sprints to the Boston Marathon. I earned a Bachelor of Science degree in Physical Education and a Teaching Certificate from Washington State University, in 1973. I'm also a certified USATF Level I Coach. The last thirty years, I've lived in or near Portland, Oregon, and still race in cross-country, road-race, and track-and-field competitions. Throughout the book, I'll share several personal experiences from the tracks, trails, and roads of my running life.

1

My Story: From Four-Year-Old Track Star to Coach

Although I was only four years old, I can still remember the day I decided to become a competitive runner. The University of Washington was hosting the 1956 U.S. Olympic Trials inside Husky Stadium. It was one of the meets the Olympic committee used that year to select the track and field team that would compete at Melbourne. After watching the meet with my mom and dad, I begged them to let me run around the track. Our neighbor, Lyle Goss, happened to be an official and overheard me asking their permission. Lyle took us down to the track, and I took off. A few elite athletes joined me and pretended to race along. Some remaining fans started cheering. I thought it was a real race, so I gave them a show by running all the way around the track as fast as I could. That was a long time ago, but it made a pretty deep impression that has been with me for more than fifty years. Since that day, a big part of my life has revolved around running fast or far, and then training for a chance to try again.

When I grew up in the 1950s and '60s, children just got together and played games and sports in the neighborhood, until our moms called us in for dinner or to go to bed. We didn't have all the organized sports and activities kids enjoy today. No computers or video games, we had to invent most of our own fun. What complicated matters for me was the fact that I was an only child and we moved from Seattle to Portland to two different towns in the San Francisco Bay Area and back to Seattle before I finished the eighth grade. As the perennial new kid, I used my speed and athletic ability to get acceptance. I'd challenge the fastest kid my age to a foot race, and I always seemed to win. With nothing to lose, I'd then race any of the older boys up to the challenge—and I usually beat them too. I played little league baseball and whatever other sport was in season, but I couldn't wait for junior high, when I'd have the chance to be on a real track and field team. I did chores to earn spending money for things most kids didn't care about: track shoes with spikes, starting blocks, and a stopwatch. I measured pretend tracks around our house or neighborhood. I made little "stadiums" in the backyard, complete with shot put rings, and high jump, long jump, and pole vault runways with landing pits.

ABC's *Wild World of Sports* was the first show I can remember that broadcasted track and field on TV. In 1962, Jim McKay launched his career as a sports announcer to new heights by going absolutely nuts while calling the one-mile race during the Los Angeles Indoor Track Meet. Jim Beatty won the race with a spectacular display of endurance and speed. He became the first man to run a sub-four-minute mile indoors on a 160-yard, banked, wooden track. It made me want to be a "miler." None of my friends wanted to run that far, so I was on my own.

Three laps around the neighborhood made a perfect mile. Mom would time me from the kitchen window, yelling out my split times for each lap and the overall time. Every few days, I'd try to better my previous time. I was a fifth-grader when Dad bet a friend, who thought he was in great shape, that I could beat him in a one-mile race.

Mr. Gilbert was a former University of Oregon basketball player and belonged to the Multnomah Athletic Club in downtown Portland. We raced on an eighty-yard, banked track above the basketball floor at the club, where twenty-two laps equaled a mile. His extra height was a

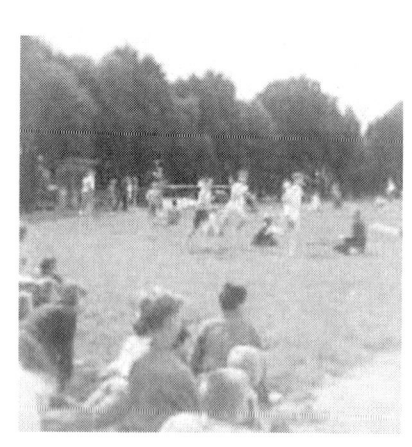

Jim in the sixth grade about to pass two eighth graders

disadvantage on the tight turns. I let him lead for the first half mile. After I got the feel of the banked track, I gathered myself for a pass just like I'd seen Beatty do on TV. I made the pass and cruised to the finish. Mr. Gilbert was a good sport. He paid my Dad and bought me a chocolate milkshake.

We moved again to a small town north of the Golden Gate Bridge, near San Francisco. Miss Bruin was my sixth-grade teacher. She was often willing to time me running around the playground during recess. My times kept getting faster, so she mentioned it to the coach up at the junior high. They checked with the league and got the okay to let me join the team a year early. Finally, I got to be on a real track team! It was just before the Marin County Championships, and coach entered me in the 660-yard run and the mile relay. As it turned out, metal spikes weren't allowed, and I had left my lighter, rubber-soled shoes at home. I decided to go barefoot on the cinder track for the sake of the team. My feet were really sore after the first race, but my desire to run the relay was so strong that I didn't tell anyone. All I remember is passing two teams and being in first place when I handed off the baton with bloody feet. The team and coach appreciated my effort and sacrifice. We were all looking forward to the next season, but my family moved to another town south of San Francisco. That meant I'd have to prove myself all over again at another school.

The summer after seventh grade, my parents sent me to the Stanford Coaching Camp for two weeks. Campers stayed in a dormitory right on campus! We had to make our bunks and pass inspections—like guys in the army. Our days were all laid out in periods just like school, except the subjects were baseball, basketball, boxing, football, gymnastics, swimming, track and field, and wrestling. All the regular Stanford University coaches and their assistants were the instructors. The two coaches who stood out the most were John Ralston for football, and Payton Jordan for track and field. Coach Ralston was at Stanford for several years and later coached the Denver Broncos. Coach Jordan became the 1968 U.S. Olympic Team's head coach. In his prime, Jordan had broken world records as a sprinter and continued to maintain a high level of fitness throughout his life, setting numerous world age-group records until he was well into his seventies. He was a pioneer in the Masters Track and Field movement. Both Coach Ralston and Coach Jordan were very inspiring men—the first to get me thinking about someday becoming a coach. That summer, I set a camp record in the mile at five minutes thirty-nine seconds, and am still proud to have been voted by the coaches as the "best all-around athlete."

Shortly after earning a starting position on the eighth-grade basketball team in my new South Bay Area school, we moved backed to Seattle. Nathan Eckstein Junior High had almost three thousand students when I enrolled. The fact that I had arrived too late to try out for basketball was suddenly not my biggest concern. I was too busy just trying to figure out which kids were okay to be around and how to find my next class. It took a few months but by the time track season started, I had made some new friends and was ready to run.

Mr. Knoll was our PE teacher and coach and the nearest thing to a drill sergeant the public schools would allow. The Beatles and the Rolling Stones had invaded America and were dominating the pop music scene. All the guys wanted to grow out their hair. Coach hated the look and thought we were going to bring head lice into his locker room. My partners-in-crime, the Walmsley twins, and I came up with the idea of shaving our heads the morning of the Seattle All-City Meet. We used the clippers in the training room to buzz cut each other and some of our teammates. When we got on the bus, coach said that some of us finally looked like real athletes. Whatever we looked like, it inspired us to run and jump our personal bests and to score points, and it helped the team win the first-place trophy.

The popularity of rock and roll music inspired teenagers around the world to play an instrument and I was a typical kid, besides my hunger to run. Some guys in the neighborhood on the track team started a band. They said that I could be in it if I got a bass guitar, an amplifier, and learned how to play. So I did—it was the first time I used anything other than sports to gain popularity. We called ourselves the Stalemates and soon started playing gigs for money. A year or so later, I joined another band called the Ultimate Weapon, which I played in until graduating from high school.

My dad had been taking me golfing and fishing since the time I decided to become a runner. I developed strong, lifelong interests in both of those activities. As if I needed additional interests, I also learned to water ski and snow ski. I continued to play baseball, basketball, and football, as well, but as the level of competition persisted in rising, it became more apparent that running track was my strongest game, with golf a close second. Those two sports would eventually take me farther than the rest.

I was not the only kid in America with the same ideas, and the competition was stiff. Jim Ryun, the phenomenon from Wichita, Kansas, had already broken the four-minute-mile barrier and gone to the 1964 Olympics while still in high school. Gerry Lindgren from Rogers High School in Spokane broke whatever records Ryun didn't attempt and challenged the world's best long-distance runners. As a skinny little high school kid, Gerry led much of the Olympic 10K in Tokyo. I believe he could have won or earned a medal, had he not sprained his ankle training in the dark a few days before the race. Both Jim and Gerry broke world records as freshmen in college. Jim set a new world standard in the mile wearing a Kansas University frosh uniform. Gerry bettered the six-mile world-record for Washington State University.

In 1966, I witnessed Gerry sustain one of the greatest individual efforts in all my years as a fan of track and field. It was back at Husky Stadium where I had first caught the track bug ten years earlier. A cold rain was blowing in from Lake Washington. The black cinder track had puddles in the middle of lane one. That forced the runners wide, adding five extra yards per lap. Gerry Lindgren decided to not hold back and busted out in his usual front-running style. His pace held steady and his lead lengthened each time he circled the track. He finally lapped everyone, including two All-Americans from the University of Washington. He broke the tape and finished three miles in twelve minutes and fifty-three seconds. It was a new American record, under terrible conditions, and only tenths of a second off Ron Clarke's world record. We could only speculate what his time might have been under better conditions on a new, all-weather track.

I would become Gerry's teammate a few years later, and like me, a lot of runners all over the country were pushing their limits to the max in an effort to catch up. There were several awesome runners my age right in the Pacific Northwest, including Steve Prefontaine down in Coos Bay, Oregon. The road to the top was getting steeper every year.

Entering my sophomore year of high school, I was a 130-lb. running back. Running up the middle into 200-lb. linemen and 180-lb. linebackers trying to cause a concussion was starting to make me think twice about playing football. Trying out for wide receiver didn't sound very fun, since my team wasn't known for throwing the ball. I decided to join the cross-country team to improve my development as a middle-distance runner. Mr. Hogel was a PE teacher, our cross-country coach, and one of the most popular teachers at Nathan Hale High School in Seattle. He recruited anyone who could run or help the team. He also made each member of the team feel like he was making a positive contribution to something special. Winning and championships were byproducts of Mr. Hogel's leadership and charisma. USA Track and Field president, Bill Roe, got his start in the sport as our team's student assistant coach.

The desire to move up the ladder created fierce day-to-day inter-squad competition. This was in the '60s; every locker room in America was plastered with slogans intended to make you work harder. The signs preached, "When the going gets tough, the tough get going," "If you're not hurting, you're not working," and "The last place you want to be is last." As a sophomore with a late birthday, and being a late-bloomer on top of that—my speed notwithstanding—I was physically behind most of my teammates. I gradually managed to adapt to the workload and moved up to varsity, but wasn't picked to race in the meet when our team won that year's state championship. I decided to train through the winter and not try out for basketball—that's how determined I was to move up the roster.

The top older runners in our school were invited to compete in Canada, at the Vancouver, British Columbia, indoor track meet. Coach was asked, by the meet promoter, if he had any milers who would qualify to run in the under-sixteen division. My late birthday worked in my favor. I ran my first official sub-five-minute mile in the preliminaries and qualified for the finals. The arena held ten thousand spectators, and was packed to the rafters! I was so nervous. My event preceded the meet's featured race between two of my heroes, world-record holder Ron Clarke from Australia and future Olympic gold-medalist Kip Keino from Kenya. Just getting to warm-up under the grandstand with these guys was a thrill. But to race ...!

They called us to the track and told us to take off our sweat suits. I looked down and discovered I had my running shorts on backward. It was too late to change them around, so I just pretended not to notice. I lost to the Canadian champion from Calgary and another kid from Washington, but we all set new personal records. My time was 4:53. A few months later at the State Junior Olympics in Tacoma, I ran 4:47. I was still only fifteen.

Being on a large team didn't allow much time for individual attention. Coach Hogel stayed pretty busy, just keeping everyone organized and under control. He talked about form, occasionally taking pictures so we could each see our form for ourselves—that was more than most coaches offered. But most of the time, he just ran us hard and let the cream rise to the top; it was up to us to figure things out on our own.

We were loaded with some really good high-school milers in Washington, at my school as well as other schools in Seattle, Spokane, and Tacoma. Some of these runners were nationally ranked. I wasn't the only runner with plenty of desire getting a good view of the leaders' behinds. Don Kardong, who went to Seattle Prep, and then ran for Stanford, and later placed fourth in the 1976 Olympic marathon, also got beat by some of these guys. (For the record, the East German who beat Don and won the race was later stripped of his gold medal for using steroids.)

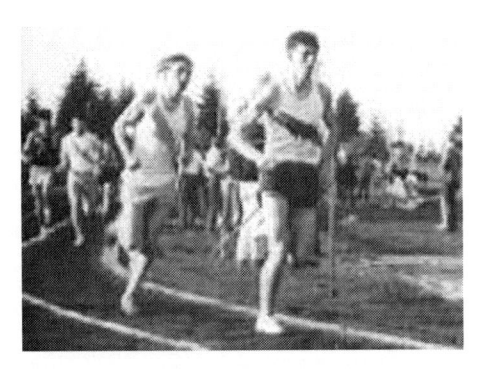

Jim leading the pack and running two miles under ten minutes for the first time in high school

Coach Hogel needed a few of us to become two-milers my junior year. Since I had the endurance to go the longer distance, that's what I did most of the season. My best one-mile race as a sixteen-year-old produced a time of 4:33. My senior year, I stuck with the two-mile. My best time was 9:39 at the all-district meet. There were seventeen large high schools represented in our district, and I placed third. In those days, only the top two places in each district went to State, even if you were faster than a runner from another district. I was crushed.

The truth was that I ran so hard in practice trying to prove something to others and myself, I was often too tired, sick, or sore to race my best in big meets at the end of the season. I would still manage to earn a decent place—but only off pure guts and determination. I won a few meets, here and there, and made it to the state cross-country championships as a junior and senior. And I fulfilled my childhood dream of running in several big meets at Husky Stadium, but I wanted more.

My teammates voted me "most inspirational" because of the way I pushed them and would literally run myself into the ground. Yet, I wondered how someone who desperately wanted to be the best had such trouble making it happen. My energy level wasn't building back as fast as I was tearing it down. To compensate, I would fall into the trap of trying to make my stride too big for the speed I was going and actually wasted more energy. **I later discovered that using a stride that is not efficient is like running uphill when your competitors are running on flat ground. I also had to learn how to balance hard effort with recovery.** Some thirty-five years later, our championship team had a reunion; Coach Hogel pulled me aside and told me it had been a mistake to let me run so hard everyday in practice. *The action assignments, drills, and exercises in this book will help you avoid some of the mistakes I made, and will teach you how to adjust your stride to the right length.*

My family spent the summers and weekends at our cabin on Camano Island, where we had five acres in the upper Puget Sound area of Washington. There were miles of beaches, trails, and seldom-traveled country roads on which to run. I didn't need a coach or teammates pushing me to train; I just did it.

Remember, I'd been that way since I was four. But that wasn't all. We didn't talk about cross-training back then, but that didn't mean it didn't exist.

My dad had been an outstanding athlete in his youth. He was enrolled at the University of Kentucky, getting ready to play basketball for Coach Rupp, when he was called off to join the Air Corp during World War II. he'd grown up in the hills of Kentucky during the Great Depression and knew about hard physical labor. He knew how it could benefit you as an athlete, getting you in shape and teaching you how to use your body in the most efficient manner. Consequently, he made sure I had plenty of chores to balance my running. I didn't get paid for the work I did at home. It was required of me—far more than what any of my friends had to do for their families. At times, I really hated him for making me finish my chores before I could hang out or train. But it was all part of his "cross-training plan." He was helping me grow both as an athlete and as a person. Eventually, I came to appreciate that.

I started making my own spending money at an early age by doing odd jobs—running a morning paper route, caddying at the golf course, doing yard work for neighbors, working for a homebuilder, and playing in the band. Later, I helped pay for college by working summers at the local cannery, and the state park on Camano Island. These jobs were good for kids. Unfortunately, today's youth in America, too often, don't seem to have the opportunity or motivation to get the same jobs and learn the same valuable lessons.

> **My breathing, heartbeat, and stride would start working in harmony: I was learning to run within myself ... by the *way it felt*.**

Some of my best training came from those days on the island where it was one stride at a time—without the worry of losing my place on the team. Out there on the beach or back road, my stride naturally adjusted, becoming the most efficient length it needed to be for the speed I was trying to run. I discovered *getting into the zone* out there and *catching my second wind*. My breathing, heartbeat, and stride would start working in harmony: I was learning to run within myself ... by the *way it felt.*

I didn't know much about mental training back then, but I was doing that too. I did a lot of visualizing, pretending I was running with and against famous athletes. When I entered meets after these periods on summer or winter vacation—when I wasn't overtraining with the team—very often I would come in with a rebuilt stride and renewed energy level. I would surprise myself by setting new personal records and beating runners I hadn't even challenged before. I was also starting to learn that some guys could post a faster time on the track, but couldn't beat me on the hills in road races, on uneven surfaces in cross-country races, or over barriers in a steeplechase.

After high school, I enrolled at Washington State University at Pullman. I had been looking forward to seeing how far I could go in the sport, under the guidance of Jack Mooberry, one of the most respected coaches in the world, and his assistant, John Chaplin. In those days, WSU and Oregon were two of the top college programs for distance-runners in the United States—and bitter rivals. Mooberry was the epitome of what is now referred to as *old school,* and he believed in sticking with the ways he had used for decades. He helped build character in boys as they matured into men who strived to reach their maximum athletic potential.

Chaplin, for his part, had an eye for talent. He was very ambitious and a hard man to impress. Just knowing that either one might be watching made you focus on what you were doing. If they happened to say something to you that was positive or helpful, it meant they had taken notice in a good way. That by itself was a big deal, with so much talent on the team. There was far less structure on the college team as compared to high school. Everyone warmed up and cooled down however they wanted. It was up to you to figure out what worked best. Some days we ran as a large group, and other days we trained in smaller groups or alone.

Pullman is a small town located in the in the southeast part of the state, near the Idaho border—about three hundred miles from Seattle. The surrounding area is known as *the Palouse,* named after the Native American tribe that once proudly raised and rode the horses now called Appaloosa. The arid and open terrain was quite a contrast to the thick-forested areas and port cities where I had lived before, but the scenery wasn't the only thing new. I had moved away from home for the first time, not counting weeks here and there at camp. And I would be starting college classes before turning eighteen.

> **Mooberry wanted me to run hard three days a week and to run easy the other days. For the first time, I was getting enough recovery on my easy days.**

Coach Mooberry was at the end of his fabled career and was known for helping individual athletes find whatever they needed to improve. He didn't waste words and didn't repeat himself, but he was willing to offer help and suggestions to anyone putting forth a genuine effort. I guess he saw and appreciated my efforts. Mooberry set me straight on a couple things, which helped me make dramatic improvement in just a few weeks. I was in awe and would have run through a brick wall for him, but that's exactly what he warned me against. Mooberry wanted me to run hard three days a week and to run easy the other days. For the first time, I was getting enough recovery on my easy days. My stride, fitness, and confidence all improved out in the wide-open spaces, on miles of dirt and country roads, through the rolling wheat-covered hills just beyond campus.

Gerry Lindgren, Rick Riley, and Art Sandison were senior leaders on the team. They had each represented the United States in the Olympics or other international competitions. Each of them seemed to be genuinely interested in helping me get better. Before the first cross-country meet in September of 1969, Coach had the four of us go out for a long run on a hot afternoon. They were men between twenty-one and twenty-three years old with world-class ability. I had just turned eighteen a few days before. They knew the route we were to run and I didn't, so I was forced to keep up in order to find my way back.

The route was a big circle around the hills and outskirts of Pullman. It went a different direction than Lindgren's famous ten-mile loop. Whatever route was assigned, Gerry was known for "running" his teammates into the ground right from the start. Luckily, he was in a talking mood that day and started slow ... for him. Rick was almost as good at this type of roadwork as Gerry. He ran high off the ground like a deer, could go far and fast with seemingly little effort. Art was an 800-meter specialist, ranked second in the United States behind world-record holder Jim Ryun. However, running long miles was not Art's forte. Fearing what lay ahead, Art and I conserved as much energy as possible and were quiet from the start. Gerry was talking up a storm, although the topics were random ... and, frankly, borderline bizarre. Rick talked just enough to be polite.

The three studs had one thing in common: they all ran up on the ball or mid-point of their feet and their shoes hardly made a sound when striking the ground. Mine were making more noise, so I made some adjustments and began to move and sound like my three mentors. After a few miles, Art seemed to give me a look that said it would be okay if the two of us slowed down. Even though I was hurting, I was in the zone and didn't want to give it up. The pace kept getting faster each mile.

I had joined the same fraternity as Art and Rick the week before. Pride wouldn't let any of us slow down. I knew things were getting serious when Gerry quit talking and was forced to think about his own stride. We were now back in Pullman and heading up the long hill toward campus. The sidewalks were narrow in the old part of town. None of us wanted to drop back, so we moved our *flying V formation* into the middle of Colorado Street. I caught a glimpse of my new home, Sigma Phi Epsilon, on the left, but didn't let it break my concentration. We were drawing stares and a few words of encouragement from students walking home from class. I'd come too far to let them pull away now, no matter how bad it hurt.

The bookstore at the crest of the hill was the next goal. From there, we could see the track a couple hundred yards away. My legs were spinning in a gear I wasn't accustomed to using for that long. I was just praying they would stop at the gate by the track. They did, and both Mooberry and Chaplin were there to greet us. I passed the unofficial initiation and earned some respect that day. Too bad it wasn't an official race. Our time was sixty-four minutes for twelve miles.

That year, there were three invitational cross-country meets WSU used to decide the team's top seven varsity members. Those earning spots would compete at the Northern Division, Pac 8, and NCAA Championships. The meets had anywhere from four to a dozen colleges or universities represented. I was always in the top twelve for WSU. To show the kind of depth we had, my highest finish was at the University of Idaho Invitational where I placed eleventh in the meet. Art, who I could only dream of beating in a shorter race on the track, managed to stay within striking distance. He had to muster all of his world-class 800-meter speed to nip me at the finish. I beat nearly all the top runners at other schools, but was the ninth WSU runner. Similar to my first season in high school, I wasn't selected to represent the team at the biggest meets, but I was again making significant improvement.

Following Coach Mooberry's advice to alternate hard and easy days, I continued to get faster and stronger. I was also starting to eliminate some bad habits in my stride. When I got it right, my feet seemed to barely touch the ground. There was little wasted energy, and it felt easy to go fast. Each day, I saw myself closing the gap on some of the best guys in the world. On some of my good days, I forced some pretty good runners to dig deep or risk getting beaten by a freshman.

As the winter days grew shorter and the afternoon winds blew colder, we would often run inside Hollingberry Fieldhouse. Back then, it wasn't heated but had lights and offered some protection from the weather. The dirt floor had enough room for a 220-yard track, with four lanes outlined in chalk. The baseball team and shot putters practiced in the middle. It could get quite dusty, and you were always on the lookout for flying objects. Saturday morning time trials were held on the weeks we didn't have a scheduled meet. The coaches would select distances they wanted certain guys to work on and run. With a stack of talent at the longer distances, and my sudden display of speed at middle distances, the blackboard had my name listed to run 880 yards (a half mile).

Gerry Lindgren had just finished his collegiate eligibility by beating Prefontaine at the NCAA Cross-County Championships, and was going to graduate at the end of the semester. Gerry hadn't run a half-mile for time in recent years and was curious to see what he could do. Coach Mooberry pulled me aside and told me to take lane one and to not let Gerry go by. I knew Gerry liked to lead, so keeping him back wouldn't be easy. Not wanting to disappoint, I did exactly as told. After two of the four laps, I noticed the usual activity had stopped—everyone was watching us. Gerry tried to pass on every straightaway, but I wouldn't let him get around. I could hear guys starting to root for me, the underdog. Gerry got to my shoulder several times, but never got by. We hit the finish line in a dead heat. The time was just under 1:56. It was over four seconds faster than my previous best, and this was on a slow track with temperatures around 25 degrees. I was in "lactic-acid wonderland" from the effects of going deep into oxygen debt, but the pain quickly disappeared. With hands on knees and trying to catch my breath, I glanced over to see a smiling Coach Mooberry give me a wink of approval.

The next weekend was the WSU Cougar Indoor meet. The dirt floor in the field house was dragged smooth. New chalk outlined the track. The baseball bleachers were brought inside for the fans. I was entered in the 1,000-yard run for freshman and sophomores.

Warming-up, I heard a familiar voice in the stands say "Go get 'em, son!" Dad and Mom had driven clear across the state to surprise me. I ran the same way I had the week before for four laps and kicked in the extra 120 yards to win my first race in an officially-sanctioned college meet.

In addition to trying to please Coach Mooberry, I was also trying to please the upper classmen in my fraternity. I didn't let coach know what was going on when those two interests collided. *Hell Week* activities took place in February, just as I was trying to earn a spot on the varsity track team. The wasted energy attempting to do both took a toll. During the week, my pledge brothers and I were allowed little or no sleep. We did ridiculous assignments that often made a mess of the fraternity house, and then were required to clean it all up afterward. By the time we finished, it was time to go to class, and the upper classmen made sure we attended. I would then go to track practice and *run my butt off*. My pledge brothers and I barely survived, but were initiated into the house. I wound up with a case of pneumonia, but I ignored the severity of the illness and continued to train and compete. Somehow my stride remained smooth and *in the groove*.

I continued to set some new personal records. However, some days I could barely walk home after practice. I started falling asleep in class and my grades began to slide. A fraternity brother started calling me Lightning, an oxymoron stemming from the fact that I could run so fast yet was walking and talking so slow. Eventually, I saw a doctor and discovered I had mononucleosis—on top of the pneumonia. I had to stop running for several months in order to regain my strength. It took time for my bloodwork, studies, and running to make a full recovery.

I finally started to regain my form during my second cross-country season. Just as I was getting ready for track season my sophomore year, I broke my big toe attempting to learn how to do a back flip for my gymnastics coaching class, and I had to sit out spring track.

Coach Mooberry's health was on the decline and John Chaplin began taking over most of the duties. Coach Chaplin more than made up for Coach Mooberry's stingy use of words, and earned himself the nickname Gabby. A former sprinter, he always seemed to be in high gear and expected fast results in everything. Using his gift of gab, he became a skilled recruiter and lured many of the world's best track and field athletes from Africa, Australia, Canada, New Zealand, and the United Kingdom to join the Cougar track team. Years later, his coaching and political skills helped him to become the head coach of the U.S. Olympic Team.

Back in the '70s, Chaplin found a way to tap into the distance-running talent pool emerging from Kenya. He'd get them over to Pullman, enroll them in school, and keep them eligible to compete for

WSU. With so much talent being assembled, he made an executive decision to work only with athletes who had met the NCAA championship qualifying standard in their best track event *prior to the start of their junior year*. I had just turned twenty the week before heading back to school. My body was finishing those last physical changes when a boy becomes a man. I had not competed on the track in over a year, and although I was in great shape, no exceptions were allowed. My days of running for WSU were over, and my attention shifted to finishing my degree in physical education and coaching.

Pullman may not be "the end of the world," but some say you can see it from there. At some point during their stay, the majority of students strangely grow a strong attachment to what we call *Wazzu* or Cougar Country. It happened to me as well. I decided not to transfer to another school. Until then, I had always gone to school only to stay eligible for sports, to impress girls, and to make a few new friends. All that changed. For the first time, I was going to school to learn. I taught myself how to balance having fun with getting my schoolwork done, and made the dean's list a few times. I earned the respect of my professors, graduated in four years, and made numerous lifelong friends.

I continued to run, but not with the same determination. Opportunities to compete were limited if you weren't on the traveling team. Sometimes, Mooberry would invite me to work out with the team when Chaplin wasn't around.

I ran with John Ngeno, the first of the great Kenyans to attend WSU. The combination of his made-for-running physique, fluid stride, and superb conditioning seemed unbeatable. I would do two repeat quarter-miles with John and sit out the third. Then I'd do the next two and sit one out, until I'd done eight and John had done twelve. My lungs were on fire after running a few sixty-second quarter miles. Mooberry and I were astonished to see John breathing through his nose, while making the sounds of an Indy 500 racecar going around the track. Apparently, he had seen them on TV. On top of that, he wasn't using his arms to run. John was using his arms to pretend he was driving the car and shifting the gears.

Three years after I graduated, another Kenyan, named Henry Rono, came to WSU and broke four world records in one season. Even if I had stayed healthy and had progressed to my full potential,

I couldn't imagine matching them stride for stride. Still, it was an amazing experience that helped further my education about the art of running and becoming a coach.

I wrote my first paper on correct running form for a kinesiology class. It went way beyond the required assignment. I was crushed when my professor gave me a C, because she said I had deviated from the original assignment. She went on to say, "This is the most complete work I have ever seen on the subject by an undergraduate student." I argued with her, but she had been teaching that class for about twenty-five years and wouldn't budge. However, she did give me an extra chance to do the original assignment over, and I earned an A for the class. My hard work paid off.

My kinesiology professor told my advisor, Dr Christopher, about my paper on running. Dr. Christopher had heard that Pullman Junior High School was looking for a track coach, and he recommended me for the job. He worked it out that I would get college credits in lieu of pay. I accepted and got my best friend, Gary Baranzini, to share the duties. He was a sprinter and, like me, had not met the required times to remain on the WSU team. We both wanted to coach and were excited for the opportunity.

Gary and I had everyone work out in one big group. That way, we could get them in shape and see how they measured up against one another. After a couple weeks of calisthenics and general running, we started slotting them into events. Gary took the sprinters; I took the middle-distance guys; and we split time with the hurdlers, jumpers, and throwers. The first meet came sooner than we wanted, but our team proved to be more prepared than the other teams. We won! Word got out around school. That's when Gary and I found out that none of the teachers at the school wanted to coach the team that year, because they didn't think the team had any talent. Hence, the reason we had the job. Funny what happens after a little organization and knowledge leads to a win. Suddenly, everyone in the building started talking about the two PE students from the college who were coaching the team. Some new recruits started to show up at practice, and the team continued to improve and win. Several individuals broke school and league records. The team enjoyed an undefeated season, and won the tri-county championship meet.

In the fall of 1972, I had the privilege of assisting Max Jensen at Richland High School about 150 miles away. We had met in Pullman my first summer at WSU when he was working on his post-graduate studies. Three years later, I needed a place to do my student teaching. Max agreed to be my master teacher and let me teach his classes, and I helped him coach the cross-country team. I ran most of the workouts with the team. This gave me a chance to work with each team member's individual strengths and weaknesses. Max really understood how to balance and blend workouts. He had a sense of knowing when runners needed to work more or work less, and when they needed to work on endurance or speed. He was a master at knowing how to bring a team along, and could get them to peak performance at just the right time. The team won the State of Washington championship and Max said that I was a big part of the team's success.

Back in the day, we were working by trial and error. And we reached many heights in running, mostly by creating environments where natural runners could ... run. But now, we know more about kinesiology, cross-training, mental training, and the variety of factors that come together to achieve peak performance—or work against it to create injury and ill health. The number one factor still lacking is information on how to develop a better stride.

That's why improving upon what we did "back in the day" means teaching individual athletes and coaches the specific things that make a better stride and how to practice those things the right way every day in training. Mastering the drills and exercises, in chapters three and four, will show you how to ... *unleash your stride and learn to run like a natural.*

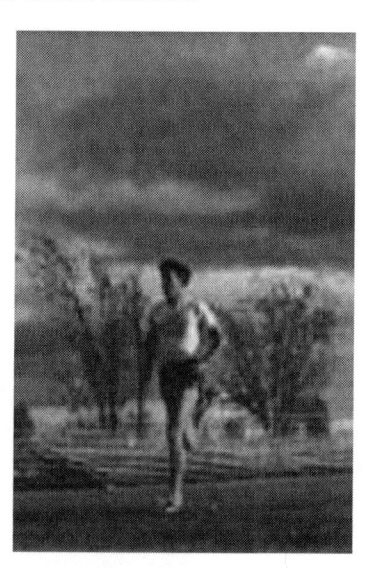

Jim demonstrating his form while coaching at Richland High School in 1972

2

The Coach–Runner Relationship: Sharing the Olympic Dream

Every now and then, a coach has an opportunity to work with a truly gifted athlete. I'm talking about an athlete who has the ability to simply move better than anyone the coach has had the chance to work with before, not to mention the potential to go to the highest level of the sport. In my case, that runner's name was Ben Andrews.

Ben was a freshman in high school the first time I saw him run. I was in my late thirties but could still run a mile in 4:40. I would go down to the high school and train with the boys on the team when I was getting ready for my own races. I had jogged down to the track one day and stopped to talk with the coach. All of a sudden, one of the runners caught my eye. He was looking around at the group he was in, and then he looked ahead at the runners in the lead group. My guess is that Ben's instincts could sense that he simply knew how to move better than the runners in the second pack. It didn't matter that he was a freshman, or the fact that it was his first day of practice with the team. From across the field, I could see the obvious—Ben wasn't going to spend any more time in the second pack.

Now, Ben wasn't the first guy to think something like this. What set him apart in my mind, which is now over twenty years ago, was what he did next. I could see his focus go inward, as he got ready to accelerate. Ben's legs started to spin faster. In what seemed like just a few strides, he made up forty yards and was settled in on the shoulder of the team captain. Ben's acceleration was impressive and appeared to take very little effort.

I turned to the coach and said, "Who is that?"

"He's just a freshman," he told me.

To which I replied, "That kid could run a four-minute mile someday … and with the right training, it could happen before he graduates from this school."

It took many years before Ben finally called me his coach. We would occasionally train together during his high school days, but always on his terms, running short, fast intervals on the track. The fact that he loved to be seen doing what he did best made the track his perfect stage. It's also an easy way for any high school coach to keep an eye on a bunch of kids who all run at different speeds. It turned out to be exactly what Ben and his coach each wanted to put into the sport.

Good athletes usually find success in more than one sport. In Ben's case, he was still holding on to the dream of being a big-time basketball player. He continued to put much of his focus on that goal. Without really concentrating on it, he soon became the best runner in the school, and shortly thereafter, began winning district championships. He had a loving and supportive family, along with lots of girlfriends who came out to see his games and watch him run. Life was good, so he didn't see the need to take me up on my open invitation of doing some endurance and stamina-building workouts together. Why should he take the risk of getting run into the ground by an "old guy" who routinely ran ten miles up and down Rocky Butte?

By his senior year, word got out about how competitive Ben was with the best high-school runners in the country—and on so little training. His talent caught the eye of two legendary coaches from the University of Oregon—Bill Dillinger, the current coach, and Bill Bowerman, his predecessor and, arguably, the most famous running coach and running-shoe inventor in the world. Dillinger had run for Oregon before winning an Olympic bronze medal for 5,000-meters. He had run under the tutelage and worked as an assistant for his mentor, Bowerman, and both had coached Olympic champions, world champions, national champions, and numerous All-Americans. In fact, more Oregon runners had run sub-four-minute miles under their guidance than at any other school, and both wanted to see Ben become the next great Oregon miler.

Ben was offered a scholarship and was off to Eugene, *Track City, USA*, and the glamour of running for the Ducks in their famous, bright yellow-and-green uniforms. Another bonus was the chance to train and race at the "temple of track and field," Hayward Field, named after Bowerman's own coach, Bill Hayward.

Ben found out in a hurry that top NCAA runners were hard to beat. He also learned that his new coaches were not going to let him make up his own workouts. He started to realize that Jim, that old guy who ran and sold insurance back in the neighborhood, yours truly, knew what he was talking about. Reluctantly, Ben began to occasionally join me on my stamina-building workouts when he was home visiting his parents. By then, he was only playing basketball for recreation with his younger brother, who was becoming the new star player at the high school.

In addition to having a smooth natural stride, Ben was a fierce competitor. Training with and racing against better athletes soon had him living up to his potential. His times rapidly improved. By the end of his sophomore season, his 1,500-meter time was 3:42. Many experts feel that is equivalent to a four-minute mile. For the next few years, Ben went through a cycle of staying up too late chasing girls during off-season, getting out of shape—and then to the amazement of everyone who knows anything about what it takes to become a four-minute miler—he'd somehow, in just a few weeks, whip himself into shape, and match his previous best times. For us mere mortals, who knew him well, it still blows our minds.

How could someone go from being so fit, to out of shape, and back again to race-fitness in such a short amount of time? What could he do if he maintained a reasonable level of fitness throughout the year? After repeating the cycle a few times, it seemed as if Ben enjoyed having people write him off, only to later have them eat their words. Looking back, he was enjoying college life, and it may have been a way of reducing the high expectations being placed upon him. Knowing the kind of sacrifice it's going to take to achieve a lofty goal like going to the Olympics can be daunting for a young man with lots of charisma and the talent to do other things. He was being pulled in several different directions at once.

After college, Ben's talent and untapped potential had some well-known coaches offering their services. In addition to Bowerman and Dillinger, the list of coaches included Sam Bell, Dick Brown, and Arthur Lydiard. Ben enjoyed receiving the attention of such noted figures in the sport. He bounced from one famous coach to the next for advice. This whole time, Ben and I stayed in touch. He often asked me and the more famous coaches the same questions about training. More and more, he found himself respecting my opinions, especially the way I would explain the *rationale* behind them.

During one of his off-seasons, when he had gained more weight than ever before, I ran into Ben and his mom at the grocery store. For some reason, after a few minutes of small talk, I looked him right in the eyes and asked, "Have you done all you wanted to do in the sport?

He said, "No."

Then I said, "Are you finally ready to trust me, do what I say—and will you quit trying to have a dozen coaches from all over the world telling you what to do, all at the same time?"

He said, "Yes."

From then on Ben started calling me *Coach*. I later found out that he asked Sam Bell in Indiana and the two Bill's in Eugene what they thought of the workouts I had him doing. They all agreed that I knew what I was doing, had Ben's best interest at heart, and that he should follow my advice.

My plan was pretty simple: show Ben without a shadow of doubt that he needed to work on building stamina to go to the next level and to embrace the process. I figured that if those two things occurred the rest would be easy. Since Ben was out of shape, we just started working out together, running five to six miles a day at a steady pace. This gave us a chance to talk. I would specifically get him to tell me about some of the races he had run—when he didn't win. I wanted him to see and admit that a lack of stamina was the common theme in his losses.

Ben's specialty was the 1,500-meter run, which is about a hundred and ten meters short of a mile. First, he needed to, once again, get back to his personal-best time. Then, if he could shave three seconds off his best time, he would be in the top ten in the

United States. That would give him a good shot of making it into the finals at the U.S. Olympic Trials. Crazy things have happened in the finals. It all depends on who is having a good day. With Ben's love of playing the underdog, he was the perfect candidate to pull an upset. By finishing in the top three, and having a fast enough time, he'd earn a trip to the Olympics.

His normal strategy was to hang behind the leaders for three laps, and then try to out kick them over the last three hundred meters. This plan worked great against less-fit and less-talented opponents. Against top competition, however, he found they could all get through those first three laps in pretty good shape and then pick it up just like he did at the end. Ben started to see that the only way to pick up three full seconds *or more* was to build enough stamina to run the first three laps one second faster and still be able to unleash his patented kick. Added stamina could also help him maintain his speed on the final straightaway, when most runners lose their form, giving him another chance to edge into the top three.

> **"When you can learn to be as comfortable pushing yourself up here in the hills as you are on the track … you'll be unstoppable."**

Like most people, Ben enjoyed his comfort zone. He wanted to run speed workouts on the track. I knew it was time to put him in his place. Ben was half my age and faster, but not in good enough shape. I knew he would have trouble keeping my pace on the big hills. So I took him to Powell Butte, where I knew the trails like the back of my hand. I led him around the easy way for a couple miles, which goes down more than up. Then we started the long and steep climb up the backside of this former volcano. First, I noticed he stopped talking. Then, he started breathing harder. Meanwhile, I was gradually picking up the pace.

When it was clear to both of us that he was really working, I looked at him and said, "You're in my world now." He told me in no uncertain terms that he didn't like my world.

I replied, "When you can learn to be as comfortable pushing yourself up here in the hills as you are on the track ... you'll be unstoppable."

Ben inherited his hate-to-lose attitude from his father. I considered it to be an asset, and began calling it the *Ted gene*. I used it to motivate him to work hard when no one else was watching. I was also counting on it to kick in at big meets, when the prep work is done and a coach has to sit there and watch like everyone else.

At first, Ben didn't really like the workouts I had him doing on the trails in the hills, but he liked what it was beginning to do for his stamina and the way he felt. He was earnestly working on improving his weakness. He showed noticeable improvement in his ability to do harder workouts and began to recover faster. But he was worried; he had been warned by others that this type of work might take away some of his natural speed. When I finally gave Ben permission to start running on the track, he found the speed was still there. Not only that, he could hang on to that speed a little longer. Ben's confidence began to grow. Once again, he started to run the times he had posted before. This time, I had played an active role.

I was getting Ben prepared to run his first true sub-four-minute mile and a sub-three-forty for 1,500 meters. To keep his interest, I told him about the series of special workouts I had designed just for him, but I wouldn't let Ben know what they were until I thought he was really ready. Out of the blue, he had a monstrous breakthrough one day. He was literally *poetry in motion*. His speed, power, and ease in movement were all truly amazing. His stamina was finally beginning to catch up to his near-perfect form.

On this particular day, he was doing repeat-200s on the track—one of his favorite workouts. Before each one, he would gather himself and let his legs naturally turn over—exactly as they were designed. His legs spun faster until he got to his desired speed. Then he would keep everything going, smooth as silk, to the finish. The top of his head looked perfectly still. He made no unnecessary movement in any part of his body. It looked like he was running in slow motion.

In reality, his balance and control was allowing him to cover ground at a rate that was swifter than world-record-mile pace. Each repetition got progressively faster, even though he appeared to be using less and less effort. He was achieving an ideal balance between the spin rate and the extension of his legs. He was definitely *in the zone*. Afterward, I told him it was time for the special workouts to begin and we scheduled the day they would start. My own dream of accompanying an athlete to the Olympics was beginning to seem very possible.

The drills, exercises, and action assignments coming up in the next two chapters will teach you the key moves that natural runners, like Ben, do so well and, more importantly, how to incorporate these skills into your own stride.

A couple days later, we met at the track. Ben was doing his normal warm-up, but something didn't seem right. I thought it was just nerves, and left it at that. Then he put on his track shoes, and did a few, last-minute accelerations up to race speed. His feet sounded heavy, so did his breathing. He looked like he was forcing the movements that had appeared so effortless a few days before. He clearly wasn't up to the task of this challenging workout.

He came up to the starting line and I said, "What's her name?"

He pretended not to know what I was talking about, since he knew we had both been looking forward to this day for a long time.

I said, "She must be pretty."

He smiled, and said that her name was Heidi.

Ben indicated that Heidi was indeed very beautiful, and although they had just met the night before, he thought she was *the one*. I put my stopwatch away, told him to put on his regular training shoes, and that he could tell me more while we did a few easy miles.

We had become very close friends, almost like family. I had known for a long time that Ben thought a berth on the Olympic team would make him rich, famous, and happy. Having followed sports my whole life, I knew of too many examples where it didn't turn out that way. Too often, athletes find themselves unprepared for the rest of their life, when their *playing days are over*. No matter what level an athlete achieves in his or her sport, there comes a time when life in general presents changes. I could sense his priorities were changing. Ben continued to train, but his focus started to shift directions as his relationship with Heidi continued to grow.

It was obvious that Heidi adored Ben, whether he was going to the Olympics or not. Yes, they were married and I'm glad to say it appears to be *happily ever after*. Although disappointed, I was happy to see his attention gradually shifting from Olympic dreams to a lasting career that would provide a comfortable life together with his new love.

Though we didn't actually go to the Olympics, I believe in my heart that we got close enough to know it was possible. The feeling is real and honest, just like the effort we put into the journey. In our minds, we were doing the work that could have easily taken us the rest of the way. It's a shame more people didn't get a chance to see the athlete Ben had become, because he was certainly ready to take on the big boys. Fortunately, he matured into a darn, good person and continues to find success in new ways. A lot of people are now lucky to know that side of him today.

> **The drills, exercises, and action assignments coming up in the next two chapters will teach you the key moves that natural runners, like Ben, do so well and, more importantly, how to incorporate these skills into your own stride.**

3

Ready …
Warm-up Exercises to Unleash Your Stride

A lot of runners seem to put on their gear, head straight out the door, and start running down the road. These runners often appear to be trying to wake up, warm up, and loosen up as they go. Even if runners wait until later in the day, it can be difficult to make the transition from what they were doing to being ready to run. I think every runner can relate to the fact that it can take a while to work out the kinks and get the mind and body working together. Masters of other activities involving movement of the whole body, such as ballplayers, dancers, golfers, and martial artists, have their own warm-up routines, and so should runners.

You need a routine that will help you get warmed up and ready to run. It's best to start warming up the large muscles around the middle first. Always start with slow movements before trying to move faster. I'll show you how in a moment.

When I was in high school, we started every workout with a series of old-fashion calisthenics. We were growing boys, and the coaches knew those exercises would improve our general coordination, flexibility, and strength. I'm convinced it was no coincidence that our teams did very well and seemed to have fewer injuries as a result of doing those exercises. We did the same routine every day in the gym, before heading outside to run. I got my college degree in physical education and studied anatomy, kinesiology, and physiology; I also took a variety of coaching classes. I was constantly thinking about how the body moved, how it could move, how it *should* move, and ways to improve performance—at first for myself, and then in general.

As a professional coach and runner, I have developed a warm-up routine for myself and the runners I coach. It is a series of six exercises that mimic movements and body positions used in running. These exercises start slow and easy, and then gradually build in intensity. The idea is to gently warm up, stretch, and train groups of muscles together; particularly the large muscles in the upper legs, butt, lower back, and abdominal area, so they are ready to move a certain way when the running begins.

Here's a little story to shed some light on why these exercises are so important. For years, I had heard coaches tell me "when you play defense, look at your man's bellybutton—he can't go anywhere without his bellybutton." When I was a student and member of the Washington State University track team, the school had a real live cougar mascot named Butch. He lived in a brick building with a viewing window next to the stadium. I started and ended many of my runs near Butch. Sometimes I would try to give Butch some exercise. He knew all about this principle of watching someone's bellybutton.

Butch and I had a game like a football player trying to dodge a tackler—or maybe more like a natural hunter catching prey. Even though he had lived in a cage his whole life, the cougar's instincts told him not to take his eyes off my middle. He also seemed to have complete control of his own middle. I've played a lot of sports over the years, but Butch is easily the best opponent I've ever faced. In four years of stopping to play our game, I can't say that I ever faked him out once. I started to realize how important it is to gain and maintain control of the midsection when attempting to move.

Throughout this book, we will need to talk about a spot in the middle of our bodies. We can't actually see the point where it starts, but it's inside and deeper than our bellybuttons. Even though most people don't think about it very much, it is the focal point of all our movement. Masters of any kind of physical activity are very accomplished at moving with this spot in mind. They practice finding and teaching others how to either locate or control this spot whenever they are talking about balance, extension, or rotation. It's part of learning how to move in the most efficient way *for any specific activity*. Whether it's throwing a ball, doing a back flip, or going downhill on skis, this spot is used as a reference point. It's been called many names over the years and in different cultures, but we will simply call this spot the *core*, as it is commonly referred to today.

Running is the fastest way we can move across land without outside assistance. The Butch story confirms the fact that we can't go anywhere without taking our core with us. It stands to reason, then, that the main objective in running should be to take your core somewhere else as quickly and efficiently as possible. How you carry or hold your core will have a big determining factor on how well you run.

The way to start building a better stride is to learn and master how to control the movements around your core. *That process involves thinking, feeling, and noticing what your body is doing.* As you are doing the warm-up exercises described below, *think* about how the movements are similar to the movements in an actual running stride. *Feel* how the movements in the exercises will strengthen or stretch muscles, enabling you to make a better stride. *Notice* the way the muscles around your core are used and come into play.

All of the first six warm-up exercises are "floor exercises," which means they are done while lying on your back or stomach. The reason the exercises are done on the floor is to begin warming up and moving in a running like manner, before asking all the little bones, ligaments, muscles, and tendons to bear the full weight and impact of running. This method also helps to align the spine and promote good posture. Many running injuries can be traced back to bad alignment causing an error in the movement of body parts.

Think about good posture as a constant goal. Good posture and balance go hand in hand. Good balance and control of your core are virtually one and the same. Maintaining good posture gives you a solid reference point to know where all body parts are in relation to your core. Consistent awareness of where your core is—in relation to the ground—helps you balance your stride.

Good posture is a function of your awareness of your bones existing in the form of a skeleton: Your skeleton supports your weight. Your muscles, ligaments, and tendons attach to and move your skeleton. The better you are at aligning and aiming your skeleton to work in the right manner, the less work your muscles end up doing, and the less tired you become. The better you become in applying the right amount of force, at the right time, to the right places, the faster you will run with the same—or even less—effort.

> **The way to start building a better stride is to learn and master how to control the movements around your core.**

Doing this warm-up routine will help you make better strides because:

- It will help you make the transition from what you *were* doing to what you're going to do (that is, *run*) by getting your mind and body working together.
- It will align your posture as you gently start the repeating action of some key running movements.
- It will teach you how to move starting from your core.
- It will help you develop balance, coordination, flexibility, and strength in the right areas.
- It will reduce your chance of injury.
- It will have you making a better stride right from the start of each run.
- It will give you a better idea of what to work on while you run, which will help you get more out of the time you spend in each workout.

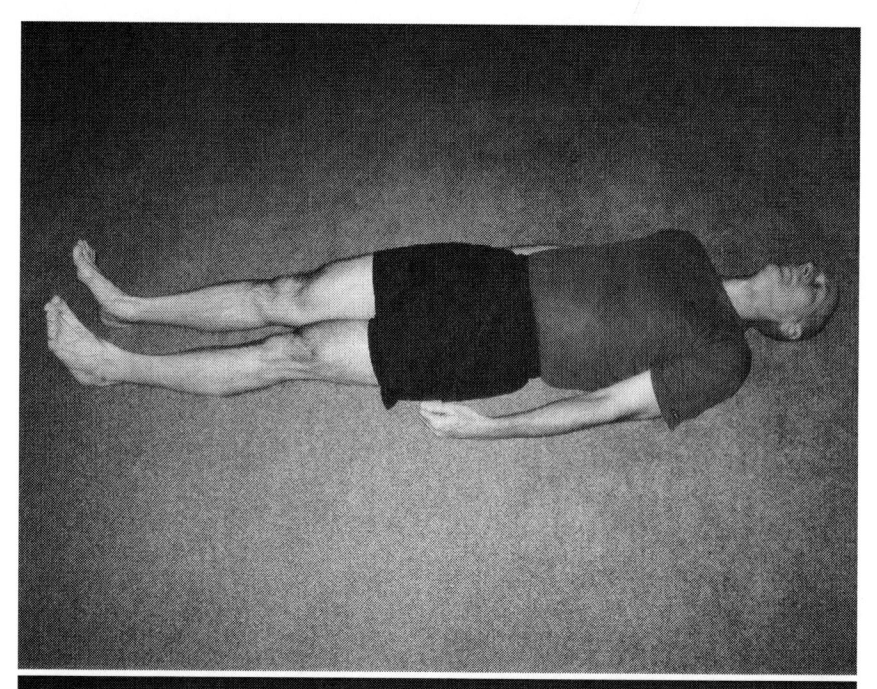

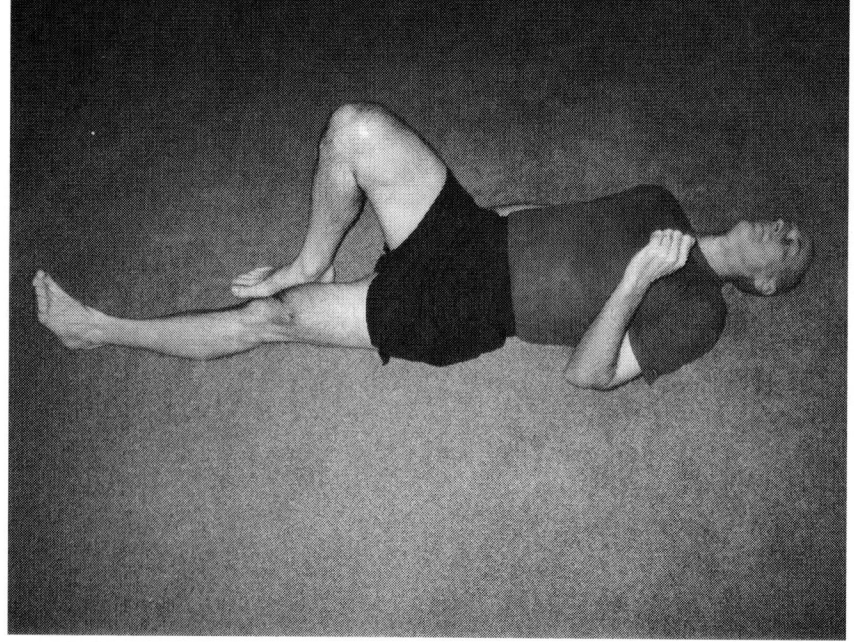

Leading Knee

The Pre-Run Routine

Exercise 1: Leading Knee

1. Lay flat on your back, lengthening from head to toe, arms along your sides, hands closed but not tight, with thumbs on top.
2. Lift and bend your left knee. At the same time, lift your right hand, keeping the elbow on the floor. Keep your right leg straight and flat on the floor, your ankles flexed, and your toes up. Continue lifting your knee and hand until your left heel is near your butt and the bottom of your left foot is flat with the floor. Your right hand continues lifting until your thumb points toward your right shoulder or ear.
3. Move everything back to the starting position. This is not a speed contest. Try to move only what needs to move to complete the cycle. Do the same thing with your other knee and hand. Notice that the muscles contracting to draw your knee up and relaxing to drop your knee down are in the upper-leg and hip area, near your core.
4. Alternate from left side to right, like running, and do fifteen reps on each side.
5. Be aware of other body parts trying to get in on the action. Keep the leg that is not bending straight with the heel down and toes pointed straight up. This position is similar to when your leg straightens underneath and behind your core when running, giving you the forward push in your stride. Most runners don't quite get to this position and as a result lose power and speed.

This combination action of bending and pulling one leg up and in toward your core (leading with your knee), as your other leg extends and straightens beneath, behind, and away from your core, is a key action used by natural runners. It provides the drive and maintains the lifted position of the core that gives some runners the look of floating over the ground.

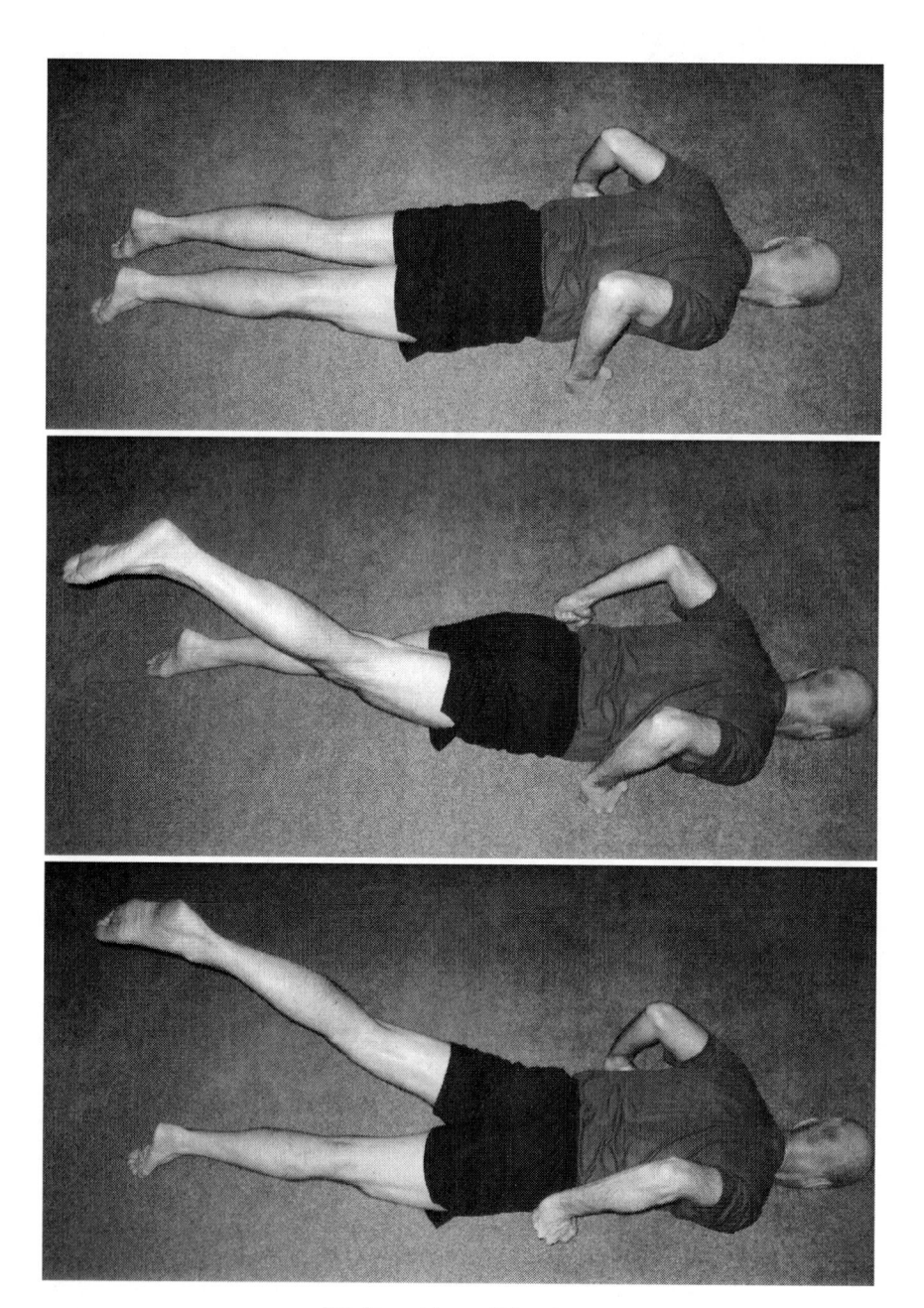

Kicking From The Core

Exercise 2: KICKING FROM THE CORE

This exercise takes a little more practice to master. The muscles doing most of the work are in the lower back, butt, and thighs. These are some of our largest muscles. Anytime they move, other body parts must move in order to maintain balance and keep us moving in the direction we want to go. Feel how one movement will push or pull something else in another direction. Feel how these movements begin near your core. Sir Isaac Newton's laws of motion are at work! The key is to *feel* where these movements begin and how you start them.

1. Roll over and lay facedown on the floor.
2. Make a loose fist with each hand and place them next to your sides, with your elbows pointing back and up toward the ceiling or sky.
3. Lift your left knee off the floor, keeping your left leg straight. At the same time, push your left-hand knuckles into the floor while lifting your right fist a little *off* the floor. Your right hip and upper leg will begin pushing into the floor. Your head, neck, shoulders, chest, and body should remain relaxed and have little movement.
4. Reverse the movements.
5. When you get back to the starting position, push your right hand's knuckles into the floor, while lifting your right knee *off* the floor—keeping your right leg straight. While you are doing this, lift your left fist off the floor a little. Your left hip and upper leg will be pushing into the floor. Even though the floor is in the way, try to get some separation between your knees. *This leg motion is similar to a freestyle swimming kick.*

Alternate sides and do fifteen reps with each side.

This exercise promotes the idea of moving your arms and legs independently, at the right time, and in the right manner. When done correctly, the equal-and-opposite action of your legs and arms will allow your core and upper body to remain still.

> **The key is to *feel* where these movements begin and how you start them.**

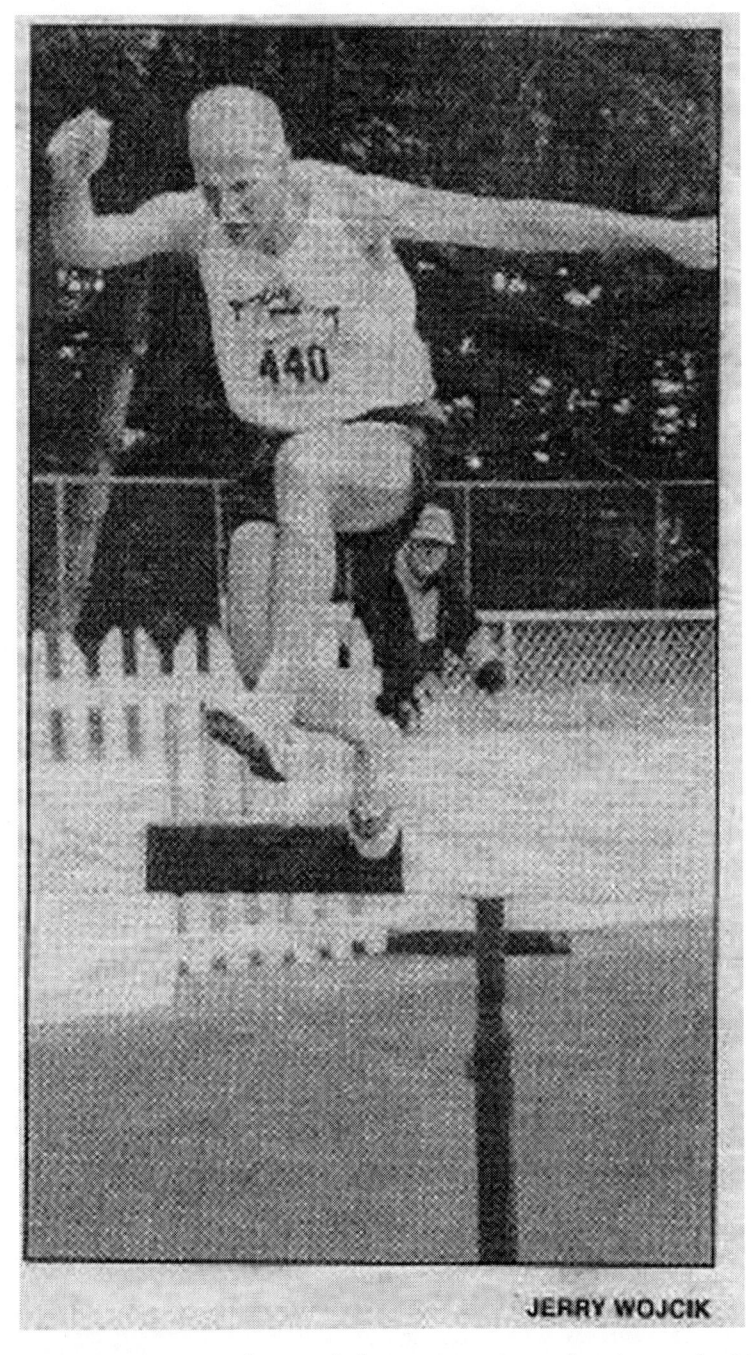

Jim, seen negotiating the steeplechase water-jump barrier at the 2001 Portland Masters Classic. His highest American age-group ranking has been second in this event

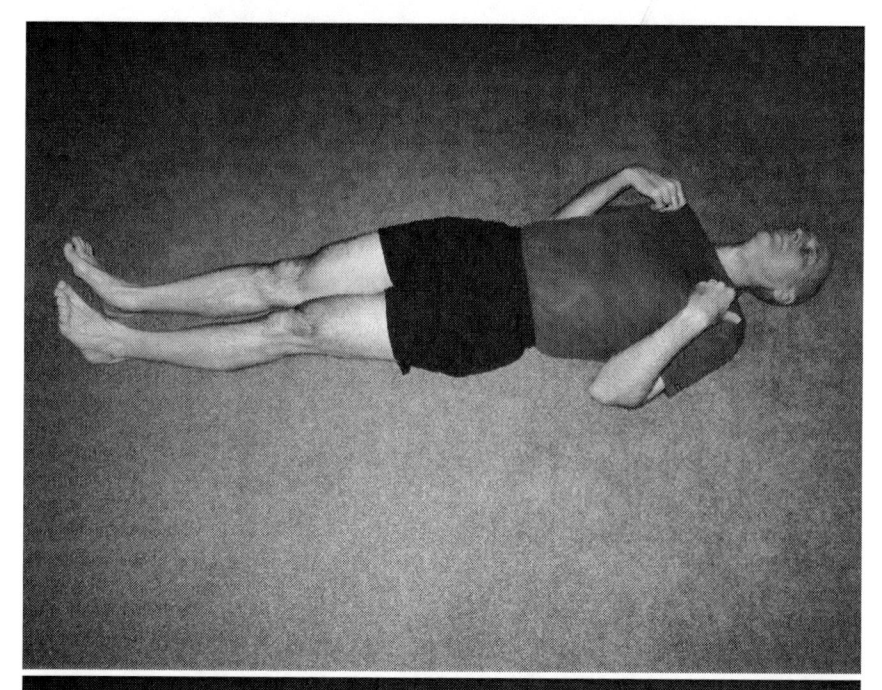

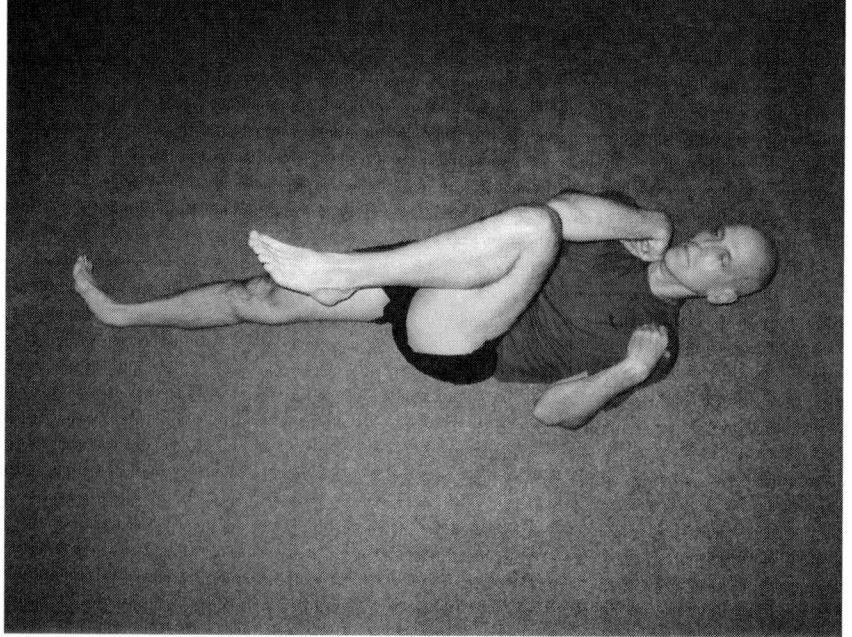

Leading Knee Crunch

Exercise 3: Leading Knee Crunch

The track and field event I specialize in is called the 3,000-meter steeplechase. It consists of running seven-plus laps around a standard, 400-meter track and jumping over five barriers each lap. In comparison to a regular race with hurdles, these barriers are thirty-six inches high and very heavy—like road barriers. They do not budge or fall down. Behind the fourth barrier lies a water pit. The pit is twenty-seven inches deep, directly under the barrier, and tapers out to track-level twelve feet beyond the barrier. The farther you jump out, the less you drop down and get wet. Needless to say, it's a tough race. This exercise helps you build strength and flexibility around the core, so you can get over those barriers and maintain good running form in between. Whether or not you ever decide to try the steeplechase, this exercise will help you develop and maintain your stride in whatever terrain you find yourself running.

1. Lay on your back.
2. To reduce the strain on your neck, place your thumbs on your shoulders.
3. Bring your left knee up toward your chest as far as you can and twist your upper body just enough to be able to touch your left knee with your right elbow.
4. Go back to the starting position and bring your right knee up and touch it with your left elbow.

Alternate sides and do fifteen reps with each side.

Bringing your knee up is more like running and jumping, compared to regular sit-ups, so try to bring your knee up more than trying to bring your elbow down when they meet.

> **This exercise helps you build strength and flexibility around the core.**

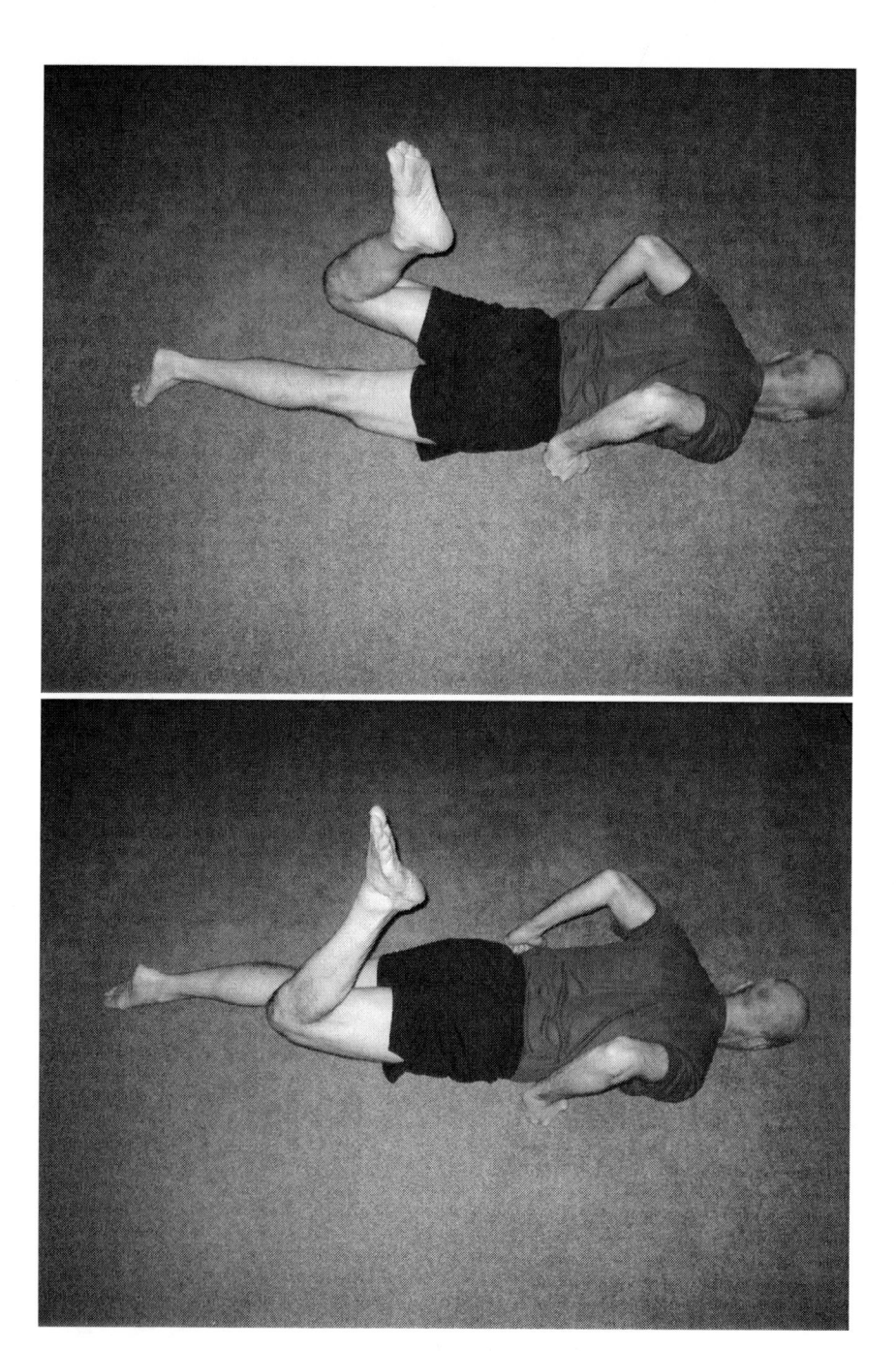

Back Leg Kicks

EXERCISE 4: BACK LEG KICKS

This one starts off in the same position as Exercise 2: Kicking from the Core, and adds another part.

1. Roll over and lay facedown on the floor.
2. Make a loose fist with each hand and place them next to your sides with your elbows pointing back and up toward the ceiling or sky.
3. Lift your left knee off the floor, keeping your left leg straight. At the same time, push your left-hand knuckles into the floor, while lifting your right fist a little *off* the floor. Your right hip and upper leg will begin pushing into the floor.
4. Draw your heel toward your butt, keeping your knee off the floor.
5. You will feel your hamstring muscles—in the back of your leg—tighten up. Your quadriceps—in the front of your leg above the knee—will stretch.
6. Hold this position for a second or two, and then reverse everything back to the start. Then, do the same move with your other leg.
7. *There is a tendency to hold your breath on this exercise. Breathe normally and try to only move what needs to move in order to complete the drill.* How's your neck? It should be relaxed!

Alternate sides and do fifteen reps with each side.

When done properly, this exercise will develop four qualities found in good runners: control of the core, independent movement of the arms and legs, strong hamstrings, and quadriceps that can stretch and extend behind. Utilizing and balancing these qualities will allow you to properly adjust the length of your stride to match the speed you are trying to run. We will discuss this in more detail later on in the book.

> **If you want to become a runner, and not just a jogger, master the skills within the *Unleash Your Stride* exercises and make them a part of you stride.**

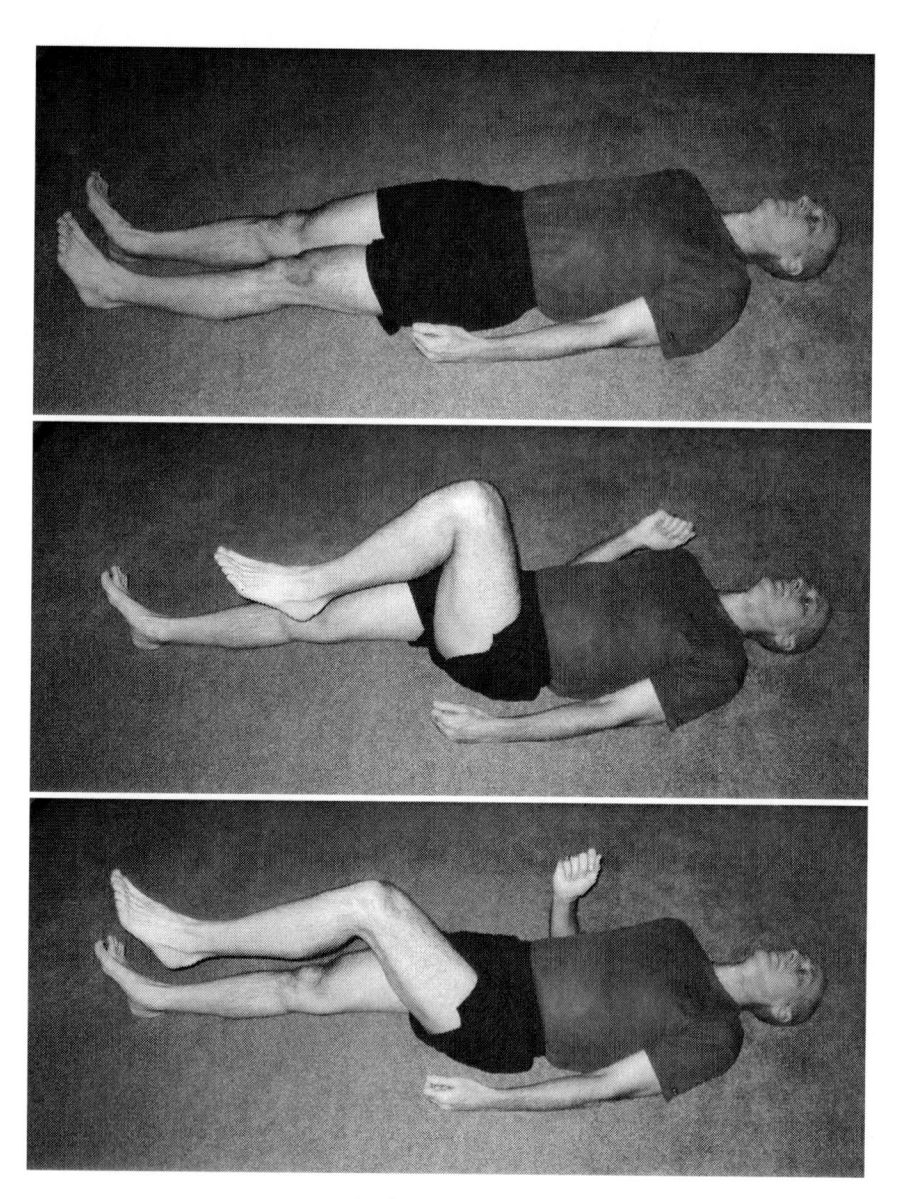

Leg Waves

EXERCISE 5: LEG WAVES

This one starts in the same position as Exercise 1: Leading Knee and adds another part.

1. Lay flat on your back, feeling long from head to toe, arms along your sides, hands closed but not tight with thumbs on top.
2. Lift and bend your left knee. At the same time, lift your right hand, keeping the elbow on the floor. Keep your right leg straight and flat on the floor, your ankles flexed, and your toes up.
3. Continue lifting your knee and hand until your left heel is near your butt and the bottom of your left foot is flat with the floor. Your right hand continues lifting until your thumb is pointing toward your right shoulder or ear.
4. Now, lift your left foot and extend your leg.
5. As your leg starts to extend and straighten, you will feel your hamstring and calf muscle begin to stretch. Your toes will begin to point up as your leg drops.
6. Notice your knee already going back down as your leg extends.
7. Do the same thing with your right side.
8. After you get the hang of this, you will feel a wave type action—from your hip, through your knee, down to your foot—building and releasing energy. The combined lever actions of bending at your hip, knee, ankle, and toes allow your forward swinging leg to move easier and faster.
9. Remember to keep your leg that is on the floor straight, with your toes pointed up. This position will create a little stretch in your calf muscles and mimics the long and extended position good runners are in when they drive or push their core forward.

Alternate sides and do fifteen reps with each side.

The key is learning when one action should begin and then giving way to the next in a smooth and continuous manner.

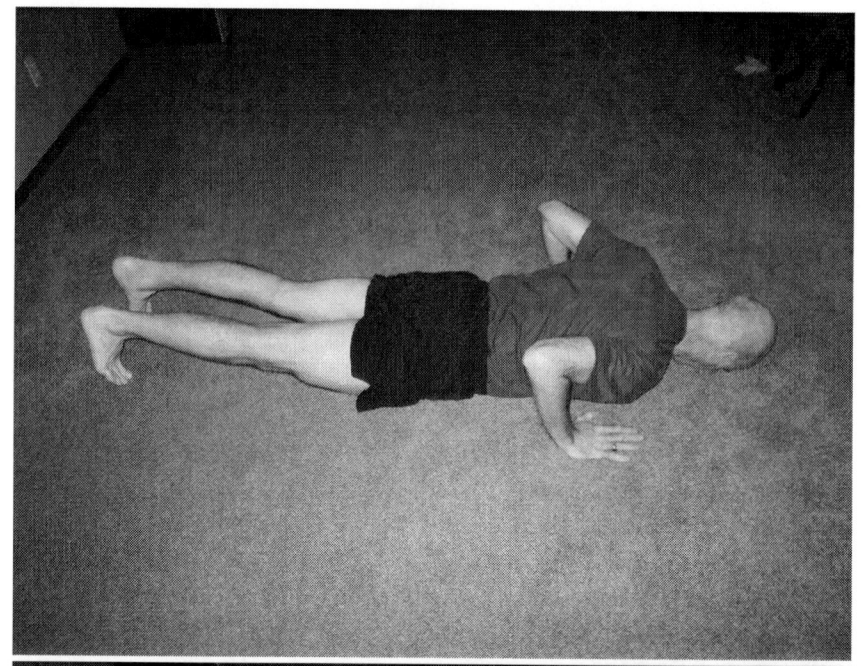

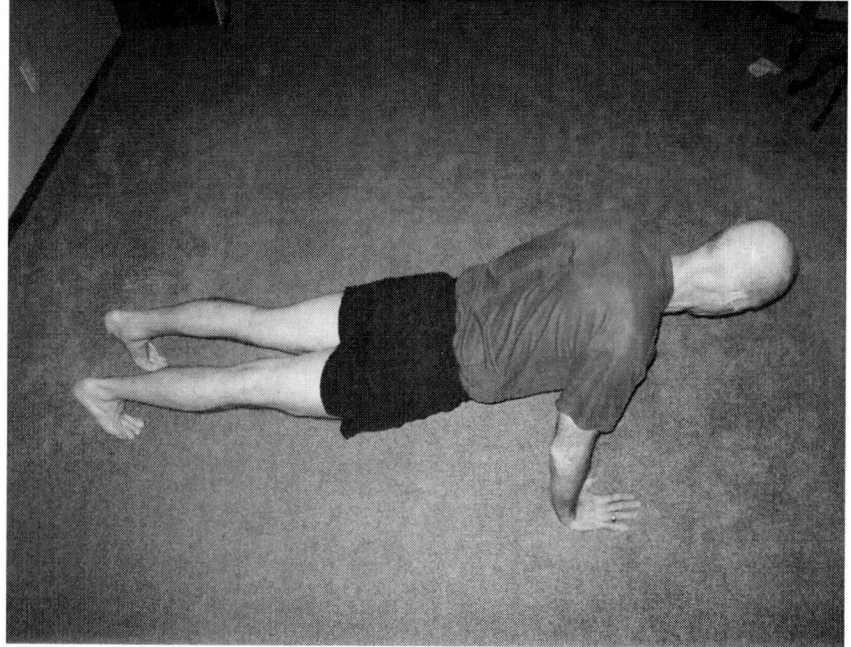

Push-Ups

Exercise 6: **Push-ups!**

Good, old-fashion push-ups are often overlooked with all the fancy workout machines available today. They still are one of the best exercises you can do for the large muscles in your arms, back, chest, shoulders, and abdomen. Lots of smaller muscles also come into play with push-ups, which help maintain core stability and posture. Too many runners neglect these areas to the point that they can barely do a push-up. If that sounds like you, now's your chance to do something about it.

- Try to do five pushups the regular way: Start on the floor facedown, hands flat under your shoulders. Keeping your back straight, push off the floor from your toes.
- If you aren't up to the task, do *as many as you can* from your knees instead of your toes. As you get stronger, get off your knees and do them the regular way.
- **Until you can do about twenty-five regular push-ups with good form, you are probably lacking the necessary upper-body and core strength to reach your potential as a runner.**

Maintaining good posture and freely moving arms are crucial to developing a fundamentally sound stride. Everyone gets tired at the end of a workout or race. If you are truly serious about improving your ability to run faster and/or farther, one very important element is learning how to maintain good form when fatigue sets in. Keep this in mind when doing your push-ups. Strive to do more with good form, but remember this is still just part of your warm-up routine.

Warmed and Ready ...

After doing these exercises, you have warmed and loosened up your muscular and nervous systems, as well as your mind, in a way that has caused low- or no-impact to your joints and skeleton. You've probably popped a few things into place and worked out most of the kinks. Your mind and body are already working together and both know what to expect. You are much more prepared to start running now with a smooth and coordinated stride. Doesn't this approach make sense, compared to subjecting cold muscles and stiff joints to the impact sustained from the awkward stride you see most runners start off doing?

4

Set ...
Action Assignments to Run Like a Natural

I have never talked with anyone who can remember the very first time he or she tried to run or what it felt like. That's because it usually occurs at such a young age, and it's hard to remember those early times. You probably got the idea from watching others, and then tried it yourself. You found out that it required more balance, coordination, and strength than you thought and, most likely, you fell down. Then you continued developing the necessary skills to give it another try. When you tried again, you either fell on your face, your butt, someone caught you, or you made it. Was it fun? Did you get hurt? Did someone see you? What was your reaction? What was their reaction?

The answers to these questions probably determined when you decided to try again. What do you think your level of determination was? Do you think you were confident and feeling ready or scared and full of doubt? Again, it's hard to say, but it's easy to see how much our actions become a series of never-ending reactions to what just happened. Rewind your memory to the first time you can still recall something unique or special about the way running made you feel. Running is obviously not just a physical activity. The mind is actively involved.

Ever since ancient times, scholars from around the world have recognized the connection between physical and mental fitness. Running is one of the most natural ways to link the two treasures. Knowing this is the reason many cultures throughout history have placed such an importance on running. In some instances, rulers have been required to demonstrate their ability to run vast distances as a sign of being able to govern or lead. Some societies have used arduous long-distance running trials as a rite of passage to measure the maturity and readiness of young adults. The fact that so much attention has been given to the act of running proves there is something special about the way the two amazing wonders of mind and body work together when we run.

What are the experiences that drew you into running and continue to motivate you today?

Whether it was a personal choice to lose weight, relieve stress, gain general health benefits, or just a competitive thing, it's important to have an idea about what makes you want to run. Make sure your commitment to running and your running goals are compatible with the rest of your life. Establish reasonable and attainable goals based on your ability, conditioning, and level of commitment. Otherwise, you may end up frustrated, rather than fulfilled, from the time you spend running.

A lot of people think they need to run a marathon in order to be considered a runner. That's crazy. Does that mean an Olympic-caliber sprinter is not a runner because he or she only runs 400 meters or less? Of course not. People need to find the distance that fits their own body type, personality, and schedule. I wish more folks would shift their thinking from being obsessed about marathons, long triathlons, or endurance relays, and concentrate on events for which they are best suited and prepared to do. They should then work out *the right way* to become fit enough to safely compete and participate in those events. Any time you make a generalization, there will be exceptions, but, in general, sprinters tend to be built with bigger and more powerful muscles than long-distance runners.

Being a student of the sport at such an early age, I naturally had my share of heroes. This usually followed whoever happened to be the latest to break a world record. I had heroes who were sprinters, jumpers, throwers, milers, and marathoners. They came in all sizes and shapes. Children learn to mimic their idols, and I was pretty good at that too. As time went on, I had quite a routine of imitations that my teammates found especially amusing. Yet, I often had no clear vision of what was the best event or stride for me. Sometimes it's a good idea to copy someone else who is better than you, especially if he or she has a similar build and has found the best technique for that build. I would try to copy just about anybody's style if she or he was better than me. Without knowing it, all the experimenting with my stride and/or techniques helped me understand the key fundamentals, and helped make me become a better coach. I learned that even though people come in different sizes and shapes, they have many similarities. That's why basic fundamentals should be followed.

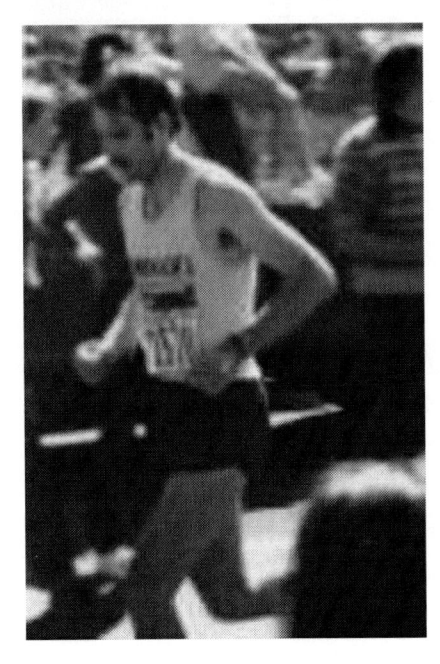

The fact that you are reading this book means you understand the value of learning from others who have already been down the road you're on and can lead you on a straighter path toward your own goal. They say that hindsight is 20/20, so I'm going to share some more things that took me a long time to learn.

After running the standard shorter races when I was in school, the jogging/running boom hit America in the mid-1970s. I started doing the popular, longer road races and marathons. I even qualified a few times for the Boston Marathon. One year, after some coworkers collected funds for me to get a plane ticket, I ran Boston and finished with a good time. However, I hit the proverbial wall in the process. In doing so, I discovered that I was neither a sprinter, nor a true long-distance runner, although I'd had some success at both. I'm a middle-distance runner. That makes me a combo or a hybrid between the two. Since I have a balance of speed and endurance, my best distances are from 800 meters up to five miles.

Jim nearing the Boston Marathon finish line

I also learned that I feel better with a little more meat on my bones. I like training for speed some days and endurance on other days, with some easy days in between. I have never been a high-mileage guy. In order to have lowered my personal best in the marathon below two hours and forty minutes, I would have had to spend much more time training on longer, slower runs. That was not something I enjoyed nor had the time to do. When I would increase my mileage—on top of the other activities I enjoyed or was obligated to do—it made me too skinny. People thought I looked sick—and often I was. I had almost forgotten the lessons I had learned in college about trying to do too much. When I'm in good middle-distance shape, though, I both look and feel much better.

As a semi-serious runner raising a young family and trying to grow my business, I didn't have enough time to train twice a day like the guys who beat me in marathons. However, I found that I could often beat those guys in the shorter road races that we all used to get ready for marathons. On forty miles a week, I was very competitive in the over-thirty division at distances up to five miles. On fifty miles a week, I could extend my competitive range up to ten miles, and was the overall winner of several local road races. The longest individual championship I was able to capture as the overall-race winner was the Oregon Road Runners Club 15K. By then, I was living back in Portland, Oregon, where I had raced my Dad's friend at the Multnomah Athletic Club some twenty years before.

The same club had an annual race on a regular, outdoor track called the MAC Mile. They got tired of the same club members winning the race year after year and decided to open it to the public. A bunch of us heard about it and ran. I beat several post-collegiate guys, and many marathoners who I couldn't beat at the longer distances. For the next few years, the race remained open to the public, and I started training for it more than for the longer-distance runs.

Running an all-out mile is a particular kind of running and requires a particular kind of training. It's very intense while it lasts. It hurts and feels good at the same time—a feeling racers come to know—but in different ways from running a marathon. I rediscovered that it suited me better and got me better results. I won my age division a couple of times, before they turned it back to an exclusive members' event. Eventually, I gave up marathons and long-distance relays altogether, in favor of shorter road races in the winter, track meets in the spring and summer, and cross-county races in the fall.

If you decide that you are not a pure, long-distance, endurance athlete, I suggest you look for a track-and-field event that *looks like it would be fun* and give it a try. There are clubs around the country for people of all ages. Many of these clubs sponsor meets with all the running and field events seen in the Olympics. I compete in some meets with participants from the ages of nine to ninety. Everything is done on an age-group basis. My personal goal is to train and stay fit enough each year to compete and strive for the running time required to earn the All-American standard of excellence in one of my favorite events. Everything is done in five-year age brackets, and the standards are adjusted accordingly. Training for these events can include a variety of activities.

Marathon training for the most part means running LSD (long steady distance). This kind of LSD might be better for you than the drug, but it would still drive me crazy with boredom. You need to decide for yourself which methods of training and which kind of events work best for you.

> **Form-faults are the result of moving something too much, too little, off line, or at the wrong time. Here's the good news: Bad habits can be corrected once you understand how to move the right way..**

Why are there so few *natural runners?*

Some people just have a knack for being able to see a task and instinctively move their bodies in the most efficient way to complete that task. The key is having the right *idea set* in your mind. That way, you know what to ask your body to do. Most of us, though, need to have some instruction. Through practice, we can train ourselves to move just like the naturals.

Running well requires total body coordination. It is relatively easy for many people to run in some basic manner, but very difficult to fully master total-body-coordination. It's not just a matter of getting into shape—fundamentals need to be learned and practiced. Since most runners don't have good fundamentals, they practice bad habits every time they run, and never become naturally good.

Running requires every part of the body to either move or be kept still. This doesn't just happen once before stopping, such as throwing or hitting a ball. The movements and non-movements need to become repeating cycles. Very few runners can do this without a few hitches or breaks in their form. These faults add up and slow the runner down. Form-faults are the result of moving something too much, too little, off line, or at the wrong time. Most people don't realize the mistakes they make while running so, day after day, they continue to practice the wrong way. They may actually become pretty good in spite of their mistakes but, just imagine the improvement they would see by spending the same amount of time and energy practicing the right way without the bad habits. Here's the good news: Bad habits can be corrected once you understand how to move the right way.

I teach runners how to find *the groove in their stride* by getting them to understand and feel the difference between movements that actually help versus movements that add resistance to forward momentum. Soon, good tendencies replace bad, and a smoother more efficient stride begins to emerge. In other words, they start to become naturals.

Understanding different running styles and how they work.

Whether you are a toddler or an elite, world-class athlete, the first objective is to gain control of your core, which requires some balance and strength. We discussed the fact that running is a series of movements and non-movements. *In other words, what we don't move—or keep still—is sometimes as important as what we move.* Once the ability to control the core is there, we need to find the best way to move our arms and legs so the core goes in the desired direction.

Most people buy into the idea that bigger is better and try to apply this theory to their stride. They try to overdo parts of their stride, thinking it will get them to the finish line faster. This is where most runners get into trouble. The ability to control the core slips away from those who try to make too long of a stride for the speed they are traveling. Coaches commonly refer to this as *over-striding*. Runners who over-stride lose some of their optimal mechanical efficiency. In other words, they spend too much energy for the results they are getting.

Most runners over-stride by reaching too far forward with their lead leg, causing their heel to hit the ground too hard and too far in front of their core. That's why runners with this tendency are called heel-strikers. Most long-distance specialists of the past and most recreational runners and joggers of today use this style. The running shoe manufacturers know this. Since their job is to sell as many shoes as they can, about 90 percent of the running shoes made today have this type of runner in mind.

The main design feature in these shoes has something to do with absorbing or controlling the forces that occur when runners slam their heels into the ground. The heel area of the shoe is usually cradled and extra thick to offer support and withstand the shock. This adds to the overall weight of the shoe. Air bags, shock absorbers, gel, and various foam-rubber materials are all used to keep the runners on the roads—in hopes of wearing out their shoes and buying more. You probably know folks who tried jogging and couldn't get it right. They were most likely extreme heel-strikers. Some of these folks hammered the ground so hard that their ankles, knees, hips, and backs couldn't take it anymore.

Heel-strikers are usually mediocre sprinters, because it's difficult to use this style and maintain an adequate combination of stride length and stride frequency. Long ago, many famous long-distance champions were heel-strikers who got tired of losing races at shorter distances. The two reasons most of them were so successful was that they were highly motivated and that they ran more miles in practice than their peers. Their strong wills and extra-developed cardiovascular systems gave them the edge. If you run more often and more miles than everyone else—and manage not to get injured—

there's a chance you can beat others with a better stride. Greater determination, along with a stronger heart and set of lungs, will win many long-distance competitions. For even better results, these runners could have worked on developing a better stride while they were working so hard to develop better lung-power—and stayed in the record books longer.

Another common unwanted movement with heel-strikers is *twisting* the upper body. It may have been cool to dance this way in 1960, but swinging your arms with stiff elbows and allowing your shoulders and hips to rotate too much won't help you run better. This action creates force in many directions, most of which won't send you in a straight line. If you have this tendency, learning to master the exercises and drills in this book will help you get rid of this habit.

A third common move to avoid or minimize is what I call *bouncing* too much. Bouncing forces the core to go up and down. The added distance of the core going up and down is like adding distance to the run. There is also the extra energy robbed from the muscles working to create the extra lifting and landing action. Newton's laws of gravity and momentum are going to eventually win this battle and will force you to slow down sooner than you wish.

The trend for most adult recreational runners is toward the longer distances. Improved cardiovascular health, weight loss, stress relief, and the lure of completing a marathon are the four main reasons most people seem to run. All of these goals are best accomplished by running at a steady pace for at least thirty minutes. That becomes a problem if you are bouncing, because it is hard to bounce for more than ten minutes. It is even harder if you are overweight. As a result, lightweight, smaller-framed runners are the only ones able to sustain this style for more than a few minutes at a fast pace. Heel-strikers, on the other hand, may not win many sprint races, but once in shape, they can often run longer distances at a solid and steady pace. That's because while they usually carry their core too low, at least it stays level to the ground and travels in a straight line from start to finish.

Isn't running the same as it's always been? How hard can it be?

Prior to about 1980, world-class runners needed to remain amateurs in order to be eligible for Olympic competition. Corporate sponsorship or accepting prize money of any kind was considered illegal for athletes. Meet promoters, however, made illegal payments to agents or Olympic officials representing the best athletes. Most of those athletes didn't see or benefit very much from those payoffs. Today, top athletes can and do make handsome incomes. The best can now support themselves until they reach their prime and maximum athletic potential. Before the change in rules, amateur athletes were forced to work a normal job in order make ends meet. They had to train before and after work. Citizens of third-world countries can now justify training and competing full-time. In the past, such pursuits were frowned upon in poor nations. Today, the economic opportunity for athletes from Africa and Asia has driven thousands to follow their dreams, running for cash as well as national pride. Although it's still a long shot, more American youths try to get college scholarships for baseball, basketball, or football, even though less than 1 percent of college athletes go on to play at the professional level, and even fewer sign million-dollar contracts.

In the early 1950s, scientists debated man's limits. The world record in the mile had stood at 4:01 for many years. Some suggested that a sub-four-minute mile was an unbreakable barrier. Others felt the effort necessary to run below that mark would risk serious or fatal damage to the athlete's heart. They argued over whether world records in other events could also be broken and by how much. Since then, more competition, increased opportunities, better training knowledge, improved diets, better equipment, and improved facilities have helped to provide answers to those debates. The phrase *records are made to be broken* is still true; records continue to fall.

The chart below lists the world track and field records, for men, from fifty years ago and the current records today. Men have been competing in all of these events since 1920 or before. Women were not allowed to officially compete in the distance events until many years later. Therefore, I did not include the times for women. It should be noted that human officials using handheld stopwatches were more forgiving in 1960 than the automatic timing systems used today. Sprinters, back in the day, could often get a jump on the starter's pistol without being detected. Modern starting blocks are equipped with devices that can sense when a runner tries to start before the gun is fired and will signal a false start. On the other side of the comparison, runners today take full advantage of faster track surfaces and lighter shoe materials. No matter how you look at it, runners and coaches keep finding ways to break records.

Men's World Record Comparisons 1960 vs. 2010

Event	Year 1960	Year 2010
100 meters	10.0	9.58
200 meters	20.5	19.19
400 meters	44.9	43.18
800 meters	01:45.7	01:41.11
1500 meters	03:35.6	03:26.00
1 mile	03:54.5	03:43.13
5000 meters	13:35.0	12:37.35
10000 meters	28:18.8	26:17.53
Marathon	2:15:17	2:03:59
110 meter hurdles	13.2	12.87
400 meter hurdles	49.2	46.78
3K Steeplechase	08:31.4	07:53.63

The athletes who are shattering records today are like their predecessors. At the shorter distances, they've had to find ways of getting stronger or having better technique. Today, the middle and longer distances are dominated by athletes who would have been fast enough to win shorter races a few years ago. Because of the stiff competition, they have had to move up to longer distances in order to have a chance of being the best. Each year, there is more competition and less margin of error. Technique and training methods have improved to a point that what we see now is, in essence, superbly-conditioned *sprinters* winning at *all* distances up to 10K and beyond to the marathon. Very little energy is wasted on anything other than driving the core straight down the track for today's champions.

The fact is, we know more about running today than we ever have. The action assignments below will help you learn how to reach your personal best.

These action assignments are designed to show you:

1. How to feel and understand where your athletic power begins.
2. How to see where you might have a tendency to lose this power.
3. How to harness more of this power in your own stride.

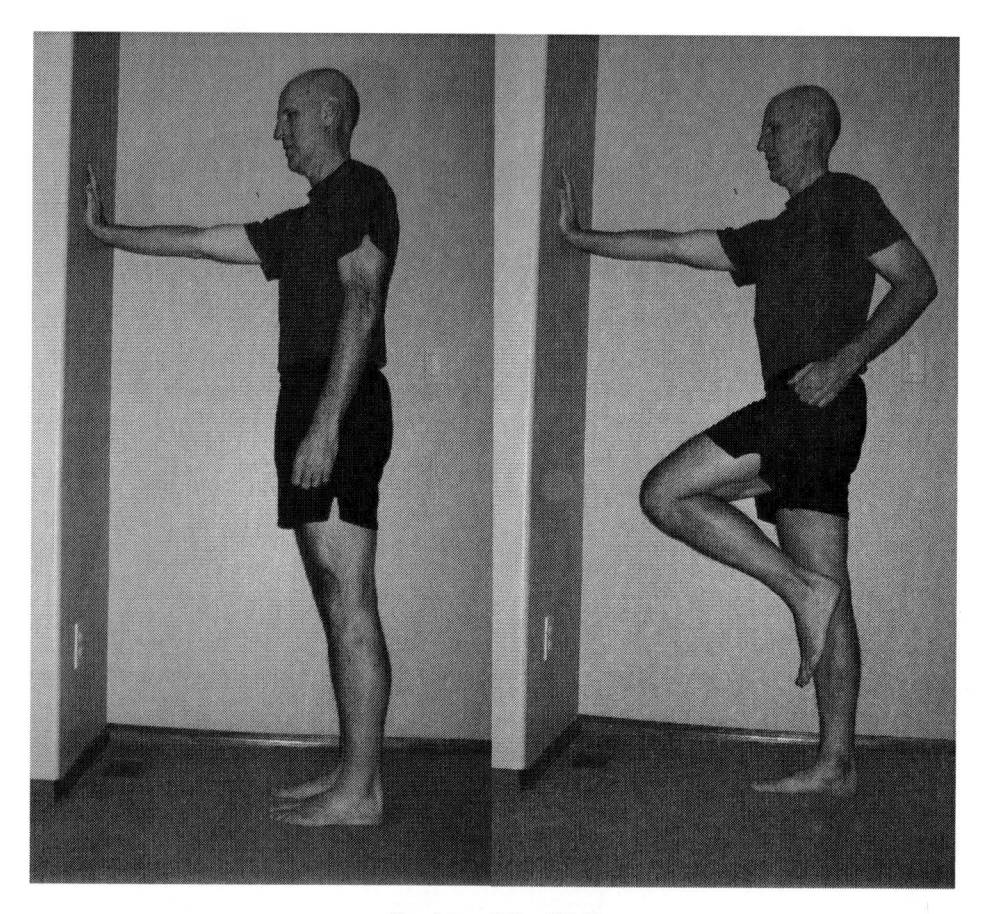

Pushing The Wall

Drills to Improve Your Stride

ACTION ASSIGNMENT 1: **PUSHING THE WALL**

This action assignment is designed to show you how to feel in your own body and understand in your mind where natural runners—and masters of other physical activities—*find their power and start to move from.* The ability to discover, utilize, and control this power source is the most important skill anyone doing a movement activity can learn. Applying this power ties into Newton's law, which states that *for every action there is an equal and opposite reaction.* In other words, the easiest way to go in one direction is to apply force in the opposite direction. This especially holds true if you push against something solid, while lined up in a good position.

1. Stand facing a wall with your feet about an arm's length away from it.
2. Extend your right arm toward the wall, fingers pointing up, and lightly touch the wall with your palm.
3. Make sure your feet, hips, and shoulders are square and equidistant from the wall.
4. Without moving your arms or legs, put your awareness in your core—somewhere below your navel—and start to push into the wall. If you are doing this right, the only way to apply force is by using the muscles around your core. Try to feel deep inside where that push begins.
5. Lift your left foot as if you were taking a step toward the wall. Some of your weight should be shifting onto your right foot and some into the wall through your right palm. This is an example of Newton's law of equal and opposite reaction at work.
6. Keeping your right leg straight, point your left knee toward the wall, while bringing your left heel up and back toward your butt; just like you did in warm-up Exercise 1: Leading Knee. You should feel more push into the wall.

7. Bend your left arm and extend the point of your left elbow straight behind you, to deliver additional push into the wall.

8. Move your toes a few inches closer to the wall and try the same moves. This is the position heel-strikers put themselves in. You can see and feel it's very hard to *push the wall*, when your foot on the ground is too far forward.

9. Now move your toes *a few inches back from the original neutral starting position*. You should feel a slight lean as you push into the wall. You should feel the weight shift off your heel to a more forward point, under the ball of your foot.

10. While keeping your right leg straight, once again point your left knee toward the wall. Bring your left heel up toward your butt. Point and bend your left elbow straight behind. You should really feel some push into the wall now.

11. Repeat on both sides until you can feel and imagine getting into this position when you run.

This is the move that naturals complete and do so well. This is the brief instance when the supporting leg fully extends both underneath and behind the core and provides the forward push. Naturals gather and use this push to maintain their forward momentum. You want to learn how to get into this position and take just what you need from each stride.

If you were running, your grounded leg would continue to extend (as in warm-up Exercise 2: Kicking from the Core), to complete the forward push.

- You know you are doing this properly when you can feel your weight temporarily supported by your bones and skeletal system. This saves energy by giving your muscles a chance to relax and lengthen, before they need to fire again on the next stride. All this happens very fast, but runners with natural strides coordinate their moves so that it does happen. Practicing it in slow motion helps your body to remember your optimal stride when you are ready to run.

You should get into this position on every stride when running at normal or faster speeds. The supporting leg should feel long and extended, even if it's just for a split second. The bent or folding leg should feel like the knee is loose as it points forward, allowing the heel to rise up toward your core. It feels like both heels are briefly moving away from each other as one heel goes down and back, while the other heel is moving up and forward.

> **You know you are doing this properly when you can feel your weight temporarily supported by your bones and skeletal system.**

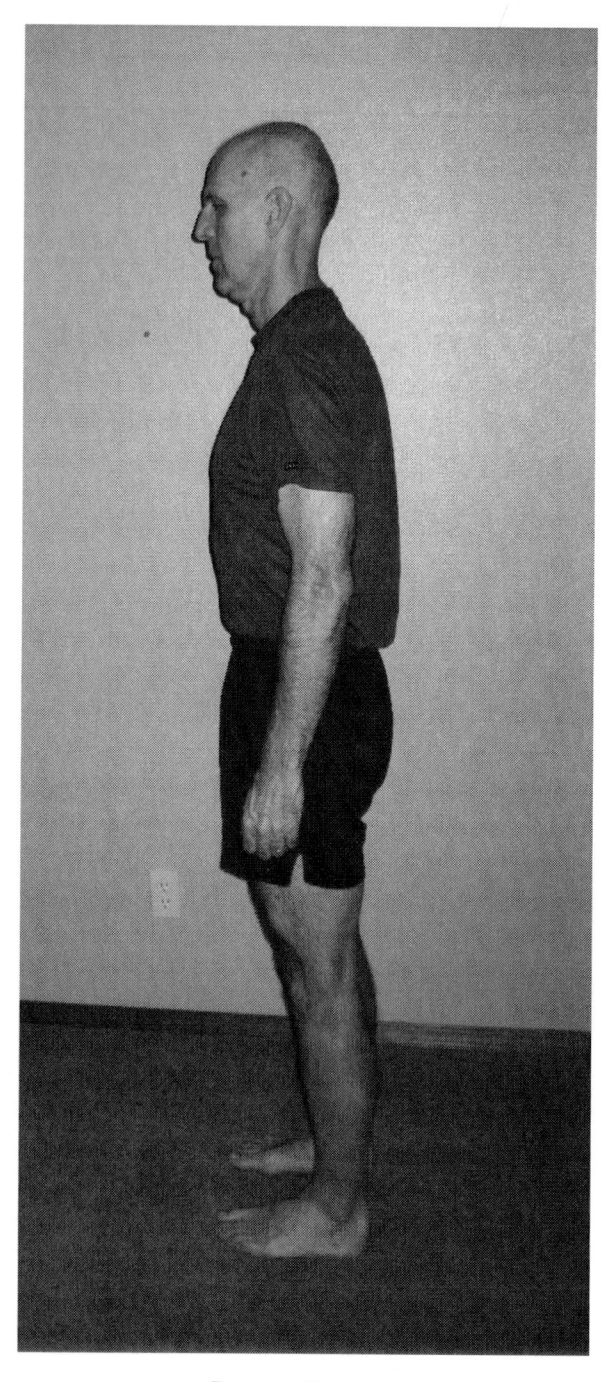

Posture Line-up

Action Assignment 2: Posture Line-up

The purpose of this assignment is to learn how to line up your body in a ready-to-run standing position. This is done by learning how to find and feel where the *focal points* in your feet, hips, center, spine, neck, and head are located. Then you will learn *what needs to move and what needs to stay lined up* when you start running.

1. Stand up with good posture looking straight ahead. Some people learn faster by looking into a mirror.

2. Center your weight onto the balls of your feet, so your heels and toes are barely touching the ground. *This is the focal point in your feet.*

3. Now feel where the tops of your leg bones attach into your hips, by slightly rocking forward and back. Your hips are supported, yet offer a wide range of motion by the manner in which your upper leg bone is angled inward—a couple inches before it goes into your hip. Find the spot where your pelvis is in a neutral up-and-down position as it pivots on the ends of your leg bones at the hip joint. *This is the focal point in your hips.* Most people have too much curve in their lower back, which makes their pelvis tilt forward and their tailbone point behind. The small of your back should be nearly flat, and your tailbone should be pointing down to a spot between your feet.

4. Your center has a focal point too. It is the most difficult focal point to find and *the most important to learn how to control.* I believe this spot is where the bottom of your spine rests; it can rotate around in the dished-out area at the top of your sacrum, located in the middle of your pelvis. It makes sense because this is where the upper part of your skeleton and the lower part of your skeleton come together. *Since your central focal point is a little above and in between your hips, it forms the top of a triangle with your hip focal points. Your true core—or center of gravity—is located near the top or apex of this triangle.* When your pelvis and your central focal point are in a neutral position, the apex of this triangle will be pointing up. Learning to find your central focal point gives you a base point by which to balance and stack your spine. This gives you the ability to develop a deeper understanding of how your upper body and lower body

complement each other and should be coordinated. *The spine should remain as still as possible when running*, so it can become the constant. As a constant, it can be used as a point of reference for all the other parts of the body that need to move.

5. *To find your neck's focal point*, follow the line of your spine up to the connection at the base of your neck. Years of sitting hunched over at a computer desk can make this area tight. This tightness will restrict the upper ribs from opening up, limiting your breathing capacity. **Check for spots that need to stretch or relax and make adjustments.** Chances are some spots may be too far out of alignment to get this right the first day. Gravity has been working 24/7 for years to affect the way you have grown and hold yourself. It takes time to reverse the process. Try to recognize that fact as you work toward improving your posture. Younger students tend to make these adjustments in posture with less difficulty. Trying to make these changes can make you sore. Push yourself to make improvements, but use common sense, and be patient if the soreness persists.

6. Continue up to the top of the neck to the atlas, or where your head rests and can nod up and down. This is the highest joint in your body and, therefore, is *the highest focal point*. When this spot is centered over all the other focal points, you are in a balanced and neutral position. If this is easy for you to do, you are way ahead of most. *Practice this alignment process every day—never take it for granted.*

7. As you get better at standing like this, don't be surprised if you notice your weight being centered over different parts of your feet. Imagine the pattern your wet foot makes on concrete. This pattern is similar to the yin-yang symbol representing the natural balance between opposite forces—in this case, heavy and light. Imagine a yin-yang symbol under each foot. Rock forward and back, changing the black area to white and vice versa as your weight shifts from your heels to your toes. The widest and darkest part of your yin-yang footprint should be across your mid-foot. **You will see improvement in your running as you learn to control this balance point.**

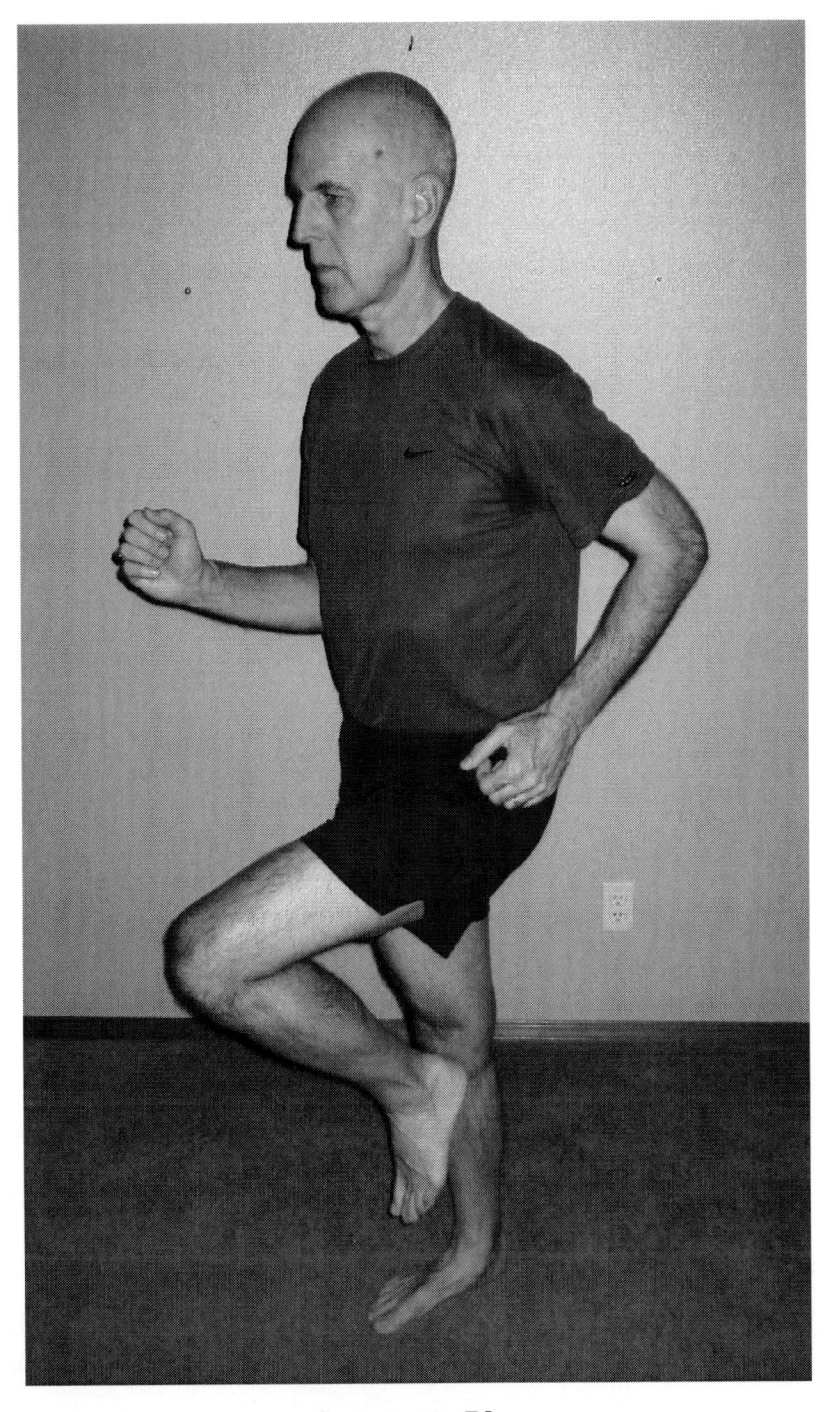

Stepping in Place

Action Assignment 3: Stepping in Place

In this lesson, you will practice how to move from one foot to the other, while keeping your balance and your focal points aligned. These skills will help you coordinate the movements between the left and right sides of your body, *allowing you to make smooth repeating strides.* Several of these movements are the same as the warm-up exercises—only now you are doing them on your feet, in a standing position.

> **You will know you are doing this drill correctly when you feel light and tall on your feet while engaging the movements.**

1. Stand with good posture and line up your focal points as in Action Assignment 2: Posture Line-up.
2. Bend your elbows until the inside of your forearms are resting next to your sides. Your forearms should be lined up parallel—like two railroad tracks—in the direction you are facing, the direction you want to run.
3. Ever so slightly, lift your heels and toes off the ground and practice putting your weight into the ground through the focal point—the ball—of your feet. Bounce a little, but maintain contact with the ground. Naturals use this part, the ball of their foot, as much as they can. *Your heels should sparingly touch the ground when running on a flat surface. Your toes are small, so don't expect them to do too much work. They are used to grip and fine-tune your balance.*
4. Shift all the weight to your right foot while you lift your left heel under your butt, and point the left knee forward.
5. Put your left foot down and repeat the same action: weight to the right foot and on the focal point; pick up your left heel; point your knee, etc.

6. Now add some arm action. Swing your left elbow back and your right elbow forward to compensate for your left knee going forward.
7. Repeat the action steps on this side ten times or until it feels smooth and you can maintain good balance. Check to make sure the other focal points in your posture are still in line.
8. Now shift the weight to your left side, lift your right heel under your butt and point the right knee forward. Repeat.
9. Add the arm action, swinging your right elbow back and your left elbow forward to compensate for your right knee going forward. Repeat these action steps ten times on the right side
10. Now shift from one foot to the other, adding the arm action when you are ready. You are still just *stepping in place*, because I want you to still have one foot or the other on the ground as you imprint the movement into your muscle memory. **Make sure you are using the focal point of your feet and are letting the grounded leg stay lengthened, until it's time to shift to the other foot.**
11. Repeat these alternating-action steps ten times, again checking that all other focal points in your posture maintain alignment.

You will know you are doing this drill correctly when you feel light and tall on your feet while engaging the movements. You should feel like you are standing on the focal point of the grounded foot as much as possible.

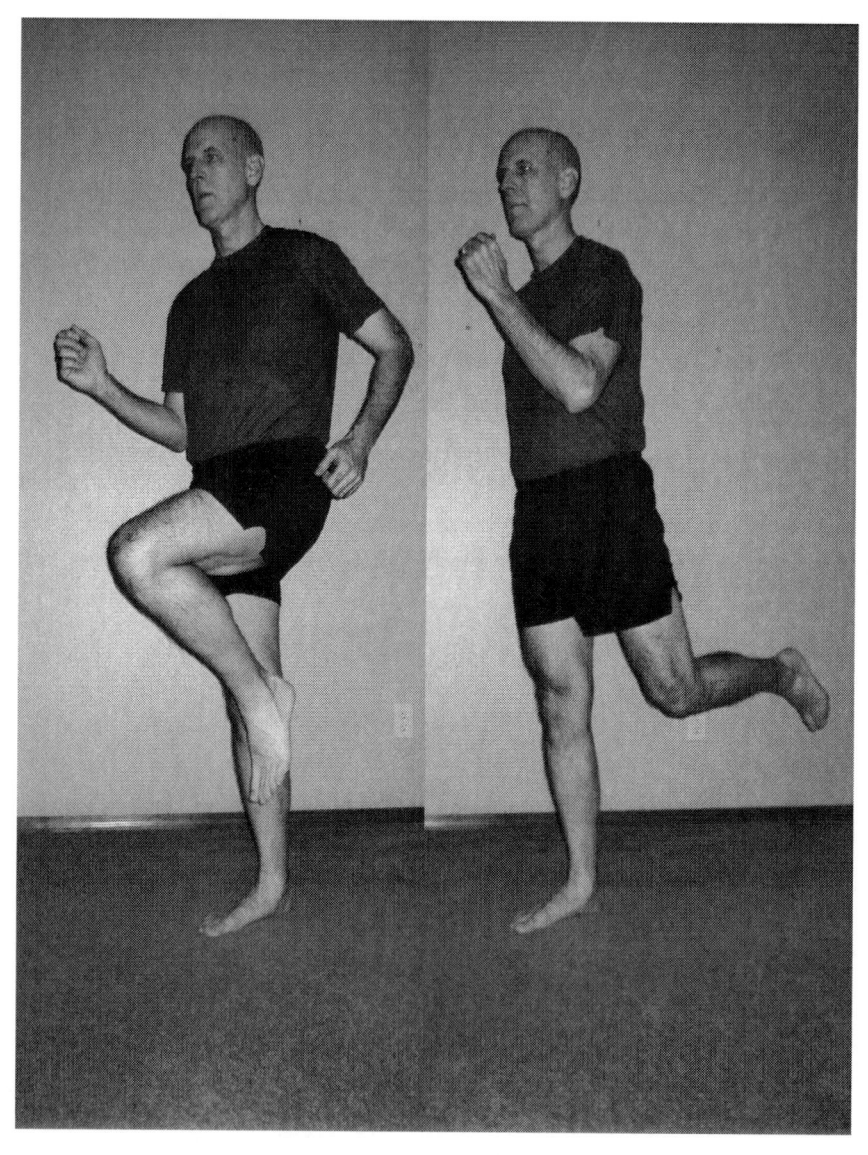

Balancing Your Stride

ACTION ASSIGNMENT 4: BALANCING YOUR STRIDE

This lesson keys in on *how to properly use the levers in your hips and shoulders.* Your arms and legs are designed to hang and swing from your shoulder and hip joints. This drill also shows you how the movements need to be timed properly in order to maintain balance in your stride. Most joggers don't know how to do this correctly, and I believe that lacking this one skill is what keeps joggers from becoming real runners.

For this exercise, you will need to find something you can hold on to—like a wall, desk, or chair if you are inside; a fence, tree, or hurdle if you are outside.

1. Stand with your left side to the support structure, so you can hold on to it for balance with your left hand.

2. Shift your weight to the focal point of your left foot, keeping your other focal points in alignment. Make sure your right arm and leg feel light and free to move both forward and back like a swing.

3. Lift your right heel up and point your right knee forward. At the same time, bend and point your right elbow behind.

4. Swing your right elbow forward and drop your right knee, letting your leg swing down, under, and behind. The focal point of your right foot should brush the ground as it passes under your core. Allow your right leg to extend behind.

5. Now, swing your right elbow back until it's pointed behind you, while lifting your right heel toward and under your butt. This will bend and swing your right knee forward to complete the cycle.

6. Repeat this movement cycle on your right side until you can feel the swing of your leg going one direction and the swing of your arm going the opposite direction (ten or twenty times). *Your upper leg swings forward and back from a single pivot point centered at your hip. Your lower leg and foot pass forward and back and also up and down because of the flexing—or hinging—of your knee. This creates a circular path or cycle that your foot follows.*

7. After it starts to feel smooth, switch sides and repeat the cycle on your left.

8. When you gain more control with the timing of the movements and can keep your balance while in motion, let go of the support and swing that arm in the same direction as your opposite leg. Notice and feel how each arm swings forward and back with the opposite leg.

The reason naturals make running look so easy is the manner in which they coordinate several movements at the same time. They allow the movement of each muscle and joint to flow right into the function of the next muscle and joint. They develop smooth and efficient power without overworking any of the muscles in the cycle.

Note that I didn't mention the knee joint as a focal point. That's because most of the time a runner's knees should be moving free, without bearing too much weight. Most runners overuse the muscles around their knees—to support their weight and to push themselves forward. That method doesn't utilize the way your leg is designed to be used. As a result, the leg muscles stay half-cocked and are overworked, which limits your power and range of motion. Learn how to swing and move the legs in both directions *from the hips and knees*. Contacting the ground the right way will allow you to use the whole leg to run. *Using your bones as levers* as well as to support your weight gives your muscles a chance to extend, relax, and contract when necessary. You will gradually start to see *and feel* which muscles need to work while others are relaxing.

Mastering these fundamentals takes time and practice. *These drills allow you to break down the running cycle into manageable parts.* As you incorporate these skills into your running, you will take your running to a new level. When you are working on something new:

- **Don't** focus on hitting faster times.
- **Do** focus on the moves you want to make.

The times will come if you do a better job of executing the right moves. The following photos show the principles you will learn and develop by repeating and mastering my exercises and action assignments.

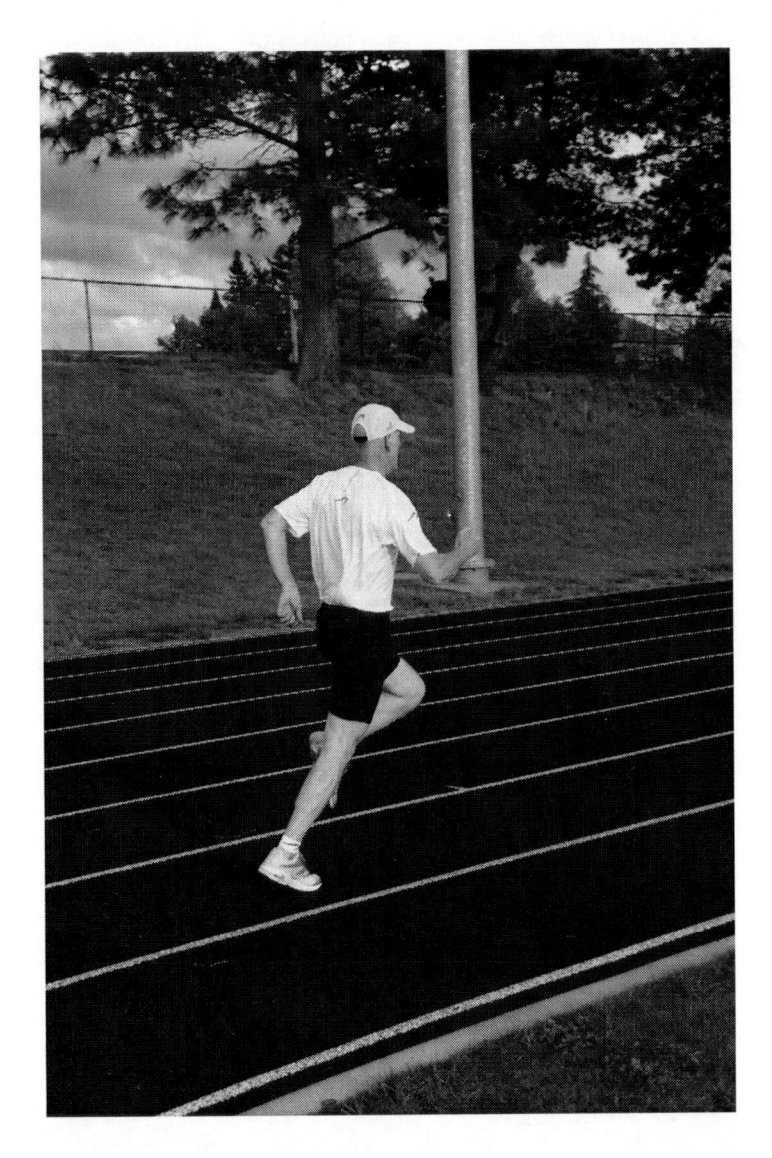

In this photo, notice how I've pulled my left heel up under my butt, like we do in warm-up Exercise 1: Leading Knee. At the same time, I'm extending my right leg and left elbow behind, like we do in warm-up Exercise 2: Kicking from the Core. Combining these principles at this point in the stride is the right way to apply power. You found the place where this power is generated and controlled when you pushed against the wall in Action Assignment 1: Pushing the Wall.

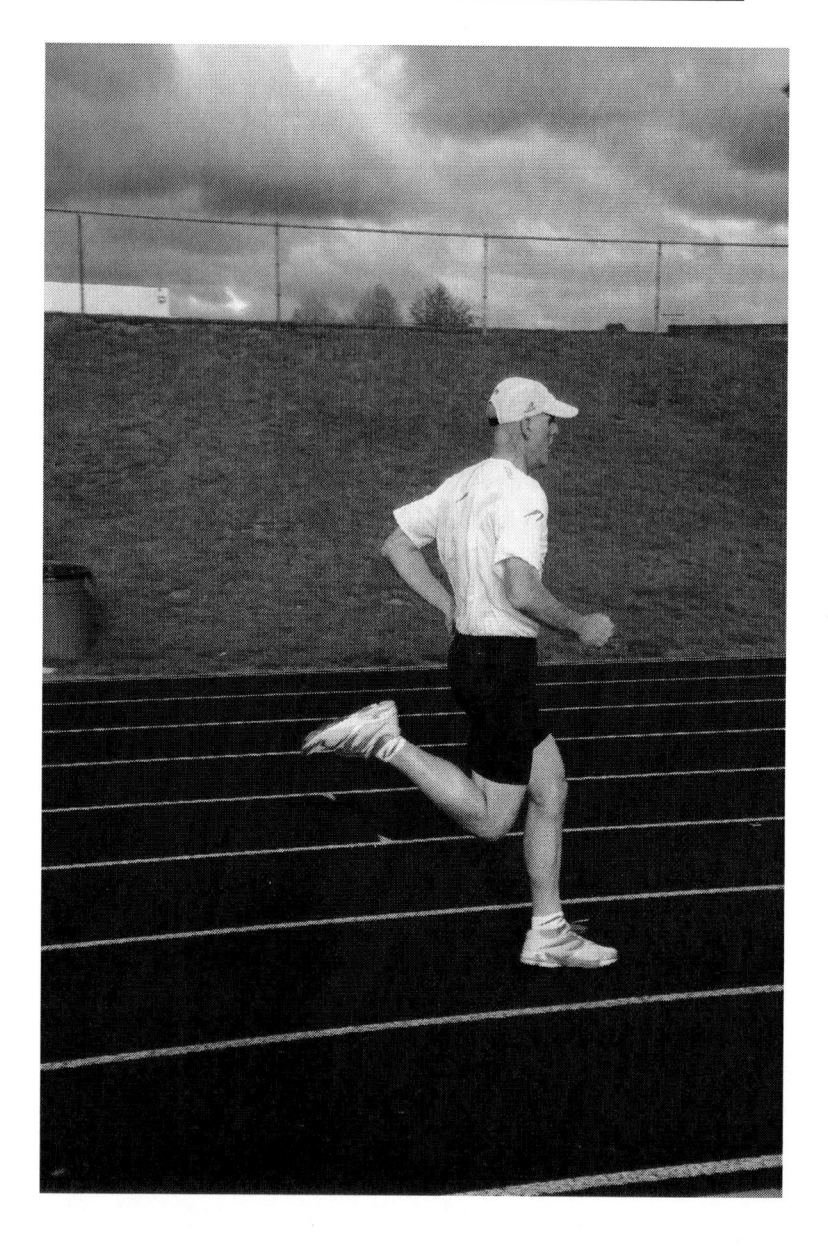

This photo shows me putting the left foot down. My focal points are all lined up, and I'm landing just on the outside of my midfoot. These are things we've discussed in many of the exercises and action assignments. Notice how I'm basically doing Exercise 4: Back Leg Kicks at this point in the stride, with my back leg and opposite elbow folded and drawn back, ready to swing forward.

Unleash Your Stride 75

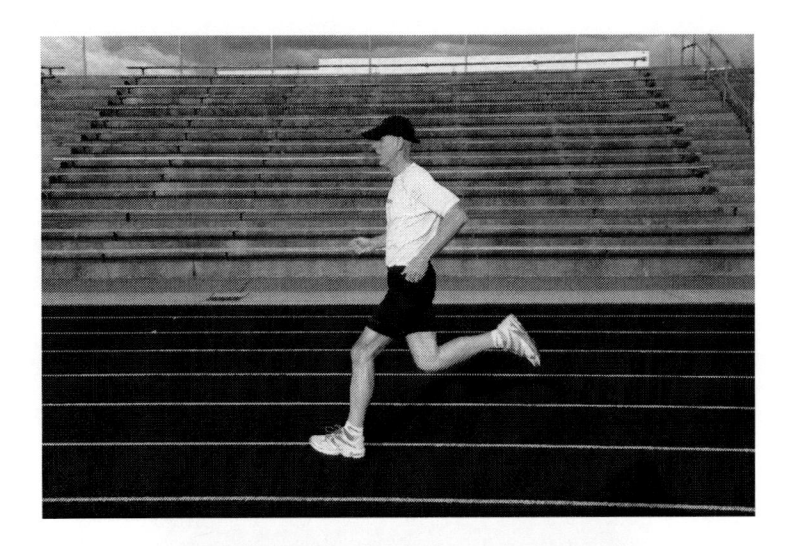

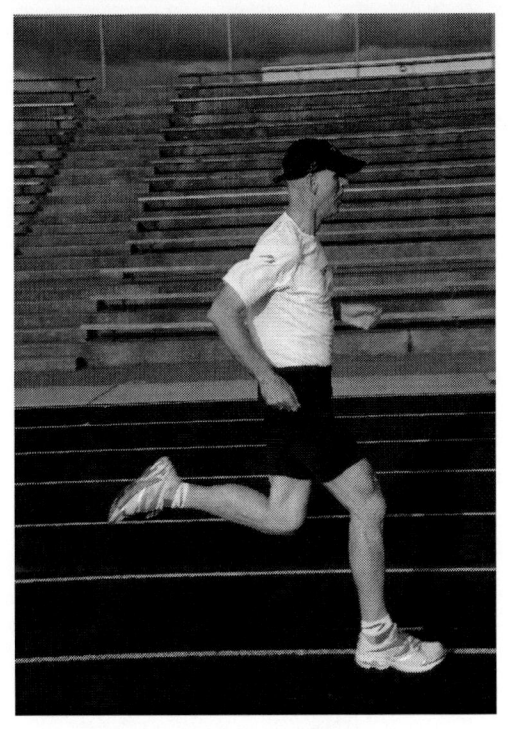

These two photos show me making nice, smooth strides and putting it all together. I'm moving under control with little tension. My knee is dropping, and my leg is straightening on the side that is getting ready to land. *This is the wave-type action discussed earlier;* I'm letting one part of my leg do some work, then letting the next part of my leg do what it was designed to do, until a full cycle has been completed. This stride building is what you are drilling in Exercise 5: Leg Waves and Action Assignment 4: Balancing Your Stride.

Notice how my spine is straight and my focal points are all lined up—in balanced, neutral positions. My arms are able to swing freely back and forth from my shoulders. My legs are able to swing freely back and forth from my hips. My core is very still and is being pushed straight forward, which is your objective when attempting to run with a fundamentally sound stride.

5

Go!
Finding the Zone

Most sports psychologists agree that it is better to concentrate on what you should be doing, rather than what you shouldn't. For instance, they say that it's more likely the basketball will go in the hoop if you think about making the shot versus trying not to miss the shot. Another example: They say you're more likely to hit the golf ball onto the green if you think about making a good swing versus thinking about not hitting it into the lake. *When you are training, think about the moves you know will help you make a smooth, repeating stride.* If you try to be too powerful, you will likely lose some efficiency. If you think about being too efficient, you may lose power. Try to find the middle ground, while remaining smooth and powerful.

The ability to focus on the linked mental and physical elements of an activity, with all distractions minimized, is what people have achieved when they enter the state known as being *in the zone*. Being in the zone—and what runners call second wind—doesn't happen every day. This describes the feeling we get when doing something fundamentally better than usual. It's hard to say whether there is really less effort taking place, or if that effort is being more effectively applied. It's probably a little of both but, certainly, being in the zone produces extraordinary results.

One such day of finding that zone happened the first time I ran in the Hood-to-Coast Relay, in Oregon. I was thirty-two and in better shape than I had been in the year before, when I had competed in the Boston Marathon. At that time, Hood-to-Coast teams were allowed ten runners who took turns running evenly measured five-mile sections, or legs.

The route went from Timberline Lodge on Mt Hood to Pacific City on the Oregon coast. Six runners needed to run three times, and four runners needed to run four times. My first leg was a stretch of highway and side roads coming down the mountain through the national forest. My second leg started from a neighborhood park in southeast Portland, went across the Sellwood Bridge spanning the Willamette River, and finally climbed up and beyond the top of Portland's big West Hills. The third leg was another mostly uphill section on small rural roads through the Oregon Coast Range. My final section went from the town of Cloverdale, on through Pacific City, finishing on the beach at Cape Kiwanda. Like the rest of the team, I was tired after seventeen hours of taking turns running, riding, and driving the van. We had a good chance to win our division, but still had two teams hot on our heels. Some of us on this team of mostly new acquaintances had already formed a special bond. I was not going to let anyone down, in spite of already running three hard legs—two of which were considered a couple of the most challenging on the course.

I got the tag from an exhausted but still hard-charging new friend, Spud Henderson, who like me had been averaging 5:30 per mile for the day. A surprising thing happened. My legs were so tired and wobbly, I quickly discovered that I could not run with anything less than a perfect, full stride. I fell into a rhythm, completely blown away with how fast I was going and how easy I was breathing. It was approaching dusk. A beautiful sunset was forming in the direction I was headed. The air was full of oxygen, mixed with the smells of dairy-farm pastures, and the fresh, salt air from the nearby ocean. Some of the grazing cows looked up, and even they seemed impressed with how fast I was moving! By the time the others had loaded Spud and caught up to me, I was more than halfway through the last five miles of the course.

My other new best friend, Nick Rocco, was now driving his Volkswagen van alongside of me. The new hit song, "Every Breath You Take," by the Police was blasting out the window. My feet were lightly touching ground, keeping perfect time with the song. The team was telling me that I had extended the lead and it was safe to slow down. I relaxed a bit but immediately felt a twinge when I changed my form. It felt better when I went fast. I yelled to Nick, "Turn it up ... and play it again!"

My form felt perfect. I put all my focus on keeping it that way, so I wouldn't—or more likely, *couldn't*—slow down. The team was pumped, knowing I wasn't going to be caught. They decided to run the last bit with me, so they pulled ahead to meet me near the finish. I was running the final mile faster than I had all day. When I got near, my teammates were too stiff and sore to match my strides. They just yelled, "GO!!!"

I finished the race and had perhaps the best single day of my running life. For the next twenty years, Nick would become my best fishing/running/sports-junkie buddy, until he passed away—too young—from cancer. Spud and I started a more social, semi-competitive running group called the Road Dogs. I also started playing my bass guitar again, in order to back up Spud and his best friend, a really talented singer/song writer named Rich Waggoner. I'm happy to say, the Road Dogs still get together and run, and the Grodie Brothers are still making music twenty-five years later.

Finding the zone feels great. It makes you want to get there again. No doubt, some days are more special than others. However, it is not as illusive as most runners make it sound. It is possible to achieve those moments on a regular basis. Learning the fundamentals and concentrating on the execution of those fundamentals is how it's done. That is how great athletes have so many outstanding performances. They deliver the desired amount of force and relaxation *at the right time*. How well you manage the amount of *extension*, *push*, and *relaxation* within your stride will determine how fast and far you can run.

Every runner uses key thoughts to lead his or her body into action. Here are the key thoughts that I use to unleash my stride and find the zone.

- Point the leading knee forward.
- Extend the back leg to drive the core forward. (When these first two movements properly occur, a runner is like a cresting wave pushing forward).
- Allow the leading leg to start dropping from the hip

before letting the knee extend. (Extending the leading knee and lower leg, too soon, causes a heel-first landing in front of the core. This releases valuable energy into the ground before the core is in position to be pushed forward).

- Then extend the leading knee and lower leg, so the whole leg can finish dropping and extending underneath and behind the core. (This is the proper way to release the wave-type-action through the leg and off the ground, so it can push the core forward in one continuous motion).
- (While the last action is taking place). Bend and swing the back knee forward in order to build a new wave of energy that can be released.
- Keep the spine and neck tall with a slight forward lean.
- Depending on the variables and situation, adjust the amount of lean, stride frequency, and stride length. Modify movements to allow for; uphill or downhill slopes, uneven running surfaces, the direction and strength of wind, or the need to increase, decrease, or maintain speed.
- Let the arms bend at the elbows, so they stay close to the body. Each arm should freely swing back and forth, both in time and in the same direction, with the opposite leg.
- Try to make these forward and backward transitions seamless and as smooth as possible.
- Let the foot land on a spot between the heel and toes when it's nearly under the core. The landing knee should be slightly bent but still extending behind to push the core forward.
- At this moment of contact, all focal points should be stacked and balanced.
- Try to spend as little time as possible in contact with the ground while still doing all the above.

Now, I can't possibly think about all the above on each stride. I might only have to think about one or two of those key thoughts to keep my stride rolling smooth. When I know something isn't right, I'll go through this checklist to find and fix any problems. Some days I'll find myself needing to concentrate on a key thought that normally isn't a problem. Usually, if I'm doing one or two of my key thoughts exceptionally well, everything else is right on or pretty close.

If you can't get your stride to work right in practice, by yourself, it's unlikely it will happen in a competitive group workout or race. That's because a competitive environment has additional distractions, such as jostling with the other runners, or being yelled at by coaches and spectators. When athletes talk about being in the zone during competitions, they mention feeling the presence of the crowd without really seeing or hearing the crowd. They will describe a sense of knowing where they were in relationship to the other competitors but were more focused on what they had to do themselves. Athletes can usually focus like this for *portions* of a competition, but all too frequently, they will allow something to distract them at a critical moment. When you are in a race, stay focused on what you need to do through those moments until you hit the finish line.

> **How well you manage the amount of *extension*, *push*, and *relaxation* within your stride will determine how fast and far you can run.**

You also need to practice what is going to happen near the end of a race, when you are really tired. As I've mention earlier, *the best results under pressure occur when you are thinking about executing the fundamentals.*

For most of my adult life, I've lived and run on the eastside of Portland, Oregon, near the Columbia River Gorge. Two enormous forces of nature, water and wind, have been working for centuries to finish the massive initial carving that took place following the Ice Age. I have run many of my training miles along this impressive river, while feeling the strong winds and seeing the flowing water continue their work. The laws of gravity and pressure dictate the path of least resistance and, consequently, the direction and speed with which the water and air pass. Both water and air have the tendency to go downhill, unless enough pressure is being applied to make them go up.

Over time, the water and wind have been working to carve the smoothest route from the higher elevations east of the Cascade Mountains, through the gorge to the west near Portland, and out to the Pacific Ocean. Today the river channel averages over a mile in width and is only one hundred feet above sea level at a point nearly one hundred miles inland. Even though it is only dropping a foot or so per mile, the river flows up to five miles per hour, as long as there is enough water upstream to provide the push. Just a small tilt or change in angle is enough to change the speed and direction of the river, similar to the way small adjustments in your mechanics either help or hinder the flow of your stride. Small differences in air pressure on either side of the mountains determine which way the wind blows through the gorge. Most of the time, the Columbia River's water and the air above it move in harmony—and in the same direction. That is nature's way.

Train yourself to move and breathe in harmony. Carve away anything that gets in the way of your making better strides and breathing freely. The key is to learn how to hold your posture and move what needs to move—without holding your breath. Your ribs and lungs need to be free to expand and contract while you maintain good arm and leg cycles. Every time it feels right, take an inventory of what you are doing—follow all your focal points from foot to head—so you can keep it going and then find it again another day.

Running barefoot seems to make runners naturally gather and align their focal points. Their posture gets better, which allows them to make a more natural stride. They tend to touch the ground with their foot more directly under their core. The impact is lighter and on a spot closer to the outside of their mid-foot. The supporting leg quickly extends behind and pushes the core forward. Barefoot runners are more likely to quickly pick up the extended leg by hinging at the hip, knee, and ankle. As the foot passes in front of the core, the leg unhinges—just like you are practicing in the warm-up exercises and action assignments. Their toes seem to be more active. When those things happen in a runner's stride, either with or without shoes, they tend to move in a very smooth, powerful, and efficient manner. Most modern running shoes are designed to protect us from our own mistakes.

Many of the today's best middle- and long-distance runners grew up running barefoot—in the rural areas of Africa. With few exceptions, the champions from these areas all seem to maintain very good upper-body posture, which remains steady and quiet while their legs and arms repeat their cycles. This style pushes their core and upper body forward in a straight line at a smooth speed. This is what *you* want.

Each year, when my kids were growing up, we would spend a week on the Oregon coast. After a week of playing with them and running barefoot on the beach, my feet would toughen up and adjust to not wearing shoes. It also made my stride very smooth and efficient. By the last day of one vacation at the beach, I didn't seem to have any mistakes left in my stride. I got up before the rest of the family and went for one last barefoot beach run. It was misty and calm, before the shift in tides. Hardly a soul was out as it was still early. At the time, I was regularly timing myself on the track and racing, so I was very aware of my pacing. I headed south for half an hour at a six-minute-mile pace. The outward half of the run felt easy, the Pacific Ocean on my right and the cloud-covered, evergreen hills on my left. On the way back, I found myself matching the footprints in the sand I had made going out. I couldn't resist picking up the pace. I felt so free and easy. It was the most effortless ten miles I can ever remember.

We loaded up all our stuff from the week-long vacation and got back to Portland sooner than expected. There was a track meet that evening at the local college. I had known about the meet, but I didn't think I would be back in time to run. Although I had just run a brisk ten-miler that morning, I wasn't tired and my legs felt surprisingly fresh. As you've already figured out, I went to the meet, and ran my fastest 5K in years—by pretending I was still running barefoot on the beach.

I'm not trying to tell everyone to run ten miles the morning of a race, or to throw away their shoes. That would be foolish. Barefoot running can be a good way to test how smooth you are striding. If your stride fundamentals are sound, you can run barefoot and run well. For most of you reading this, either the climate, the area you run, your current stride, or the softness of your feet won't allow you to run without some protection. After cutting myself too many times on broken glass, shells, and debris, I now wear aqua-socks for protection on the few occasions I do run at the beach. When I want that barefoot feel, and can't run on the beach, I wear aqua-socks on grass playgrounds, or lightweight racing shoes on a track. I try to concentrate on lining up my focal points. Then I let my legs and arms swing and spin so that I'm pushing forward with little resistance. I try to relax anything that feels tight and adjust anything that is out of time or working more than it should—all the things you should be doing in your regular training shoes.

6

Cooling Down— The Importance of Rest and Deciding What's Next

All runners should be in good general health and use common sense before making the final decision to run. They should ask themselves if they are up to the task of today's workout or not. Before NASA launches a rocket into space, they always have a final checklist that makes sure all systems are ready to go.

You should know after your warm-up if you are ready and set to go. If your energy is too low or you are feeling the start of a cough or a cold, is it wise to run? You have to ask yourself whether you would gain more from doing a workout or taking a day off. If you have sore muscles or a slight injury, will the workout make the problem better or worse? Even if you are following a designed workout plan, from either a book or coach, there are days when workouts need to be altered for your progress toward your long-term goals as well as your overall good. If you are having doubts as to whether you will be able to run with a smooth, fundamentally sound stride, you can perhaps do an alternative form of exercise until things get better. If you begin a workout with the hope that things loosen up and then they don't, use common sense and make the right decision about what to do next. Adapting your stride mechanics to counteract being too sore to do it the right way is a mistake. This will often lead to a more serious injury and setbacks. If the training guide you are using calls for a run that is longer or more intense than normal and you do not feel up for it that day, go easy or take the day off. Rest, recover, and be sure you are ready, before trying a big workout or a race. Some workouts require more energy and, consequently, more recovery time than other workouts. The amount of energy spent, along with the amount of energy you had before starting the workout, will determine how long it will take you to recover to a normal or even improved level of energy.

> **Remember, you didn't get out of shape in one day, so don't expect to become fit in only a day or two.**

Most runners have competitive egos. Many will try to speed up the process of getting in shape by moving on to a more advanced training level before they are ready. The temptation of running too much can be hard to resist. I designed the following charts to help runners decide how far and how often to run. The average runner may not have the time or the desire to run seven days a week. This schedule incorporates two principles that virtually all successful coaches utilize in some manner. The first is known as the *hard day/easy day theory*. Harder days of running are followed by a rest day or an easier running day. The second theory is the *incline sawtooth method*. Training volume progressively builds over time and then drops back down before the next buildup. In this case the progressive buildup takes three weeks followed by a lighter week of running. Both theories are based on scientific studies bearing evidence that the human body will adapt to increasing workloads, but will eventually breakdown if pushed too hard without receiving an adequate chance to recover. This schedule calls for running every other day for the first two weeks. The schedule shifts to two days of running followed by a rest day in the third and fourth weeks. In the fifth and sixth weeks the plan alternates between periods of running three days in a row followed by a rest day and then two days of running. In the seventh and eighth weeks, the schedule returns to two days of running followed by a rest day. The fourth, eighth, and twelfth weeks have three days of rest and therefore less volume of running than the week before. **The weeks with extra rest are an important part of the training process. They give your body and**

mind the necessary time to adapt and prepare for either a race or a more intense period of training.

Most road races and track meets are now measured in kilometers or meters. The unit of measurement used in the first chart is kilometers (k). A kilometer is one thousand meters. One kilometer is 62% or just a little less than 5/8 of a mile. That means a runner averaging eight minutes per mile will cover one kilometer in about five minutes. Use this formula if you run at this pace and don't have a way to accurately measure your routes. (1unit= 5 minutes or 1k).

			Basic Training Guide Measured in Kilometers					
Week	Sun	Mon	Tue	Wed	Thru	Fri	Sat	Total (k)
1	3	Rest	4	Rest	3	Rest	5	15
2	3	Rest	4	Rest	5	Rest	5	17
3	4	Rest	5	3	Rest	3	5	20
4	Rest	5	4	Rest	5	4	Rest	18
5	6	Rest	3	5	3	Rest	6	23
6	4	Rest	4	6	4	Rest	7	25
7	5	Rest	6	4	Rest	4	8	27
8	Rest	6	4	Rest	6	4	Rest	20
9	8	Rest	4	6	4	Rest	7	29
10	6	Rest	7	5	7	Rest	8	33
11	6	Rest	8	4	8	Rest	9	35
12	Rest	8	4	Rest	8	4	Rest	24

Remember, the charts are merely guides and can be modified if you follow the principles upon which they are based. If you prefer to measure the distance you run in miles (m), use the chart below as your guide.

Week	Sun	Mon	Tue	Wed	Thru	Fri	Sat	Total (m)
1	2	Rest	2.5	Rest	2	Rest	3	9.5
2	2	Rest	2.5	Rest	3	Rest	3	10.5
3	2.5	Rest	3	2	Rest	2	3	12.5
4	Rest	3	2.5	Rest	3	2.5	Rest	11
5	3.5	Rest	2	3	2	Rest	3.5	14
6	2.5	Rest	2.5	3.5	2.5	Rest	4	15
7	3	Rest	3.5	2.5	Rest	2.5	5	16.5
8	Rest	3.5	2.5	Rest	3.5	2.5	Rest	12
9	5	Rest	2.5	3.5	2.5	Rest	4	17.5
10	3.5	Rest	4	3	4	Rest	5	19.5
11	3.5	Rest	5	2.5	5	Rest	5.5	21.5
12	Rest	5	2.5	Rest	5	2.5	Rest	15

Basic Training Guide Measured in Miles

Following either chart as a training guide will help you build a base level of fitness. Every workout should begin with the, *Unleash Your Stride/Learn to Run Like a Natural,* warm-up exercise routine. Start your runs easy until you are fully warmed-up. This will take five to ten minutes. Maintain a steady pace that's not too fast or too slow in the middle. Ease up and cool yourself down the last five minutes of each run. You should be adequately prepared to complete a 10K road race or ready to join most high school cross country/

track teams after finishing this twelve week cycle. If you are joining a team, the coach will appreciate your pre-season conditioning and will be able to get your specialized training started sooner for your specific event. If you are an adult with a basic goal of maintaining a good recreational fitness level, repeating weeks 9-12 is all you need to do. You can feel confident joining friends for social runs or participating in occasional road races up to 10K.

Make copies of the next chart to plan your own workouts, monitor your progress, and record your results.

Personal Training Guide

Week	Sun	Mon	Tue	Wed	Thru	Fri	Sat	Total
1								
2								
3								
4								
5								
6								
7								
8								
9								
10								
11								
12								

If your goal is to run a faster 10K, gradually increase the distance you run. You will be training for an event that demands more endurance than speed. Start by adding one to two units of time/distance to your Saturday runs until you reach 15K or 9.3 miles. Finishing a 10K will no longer be a problem since your long runs will be reaching 150% of your racing distance. You can keep boosting your four week cycles by adding one unit to the other runs until you've reached the level you wish to maintain. This will give you two ways to sensibly increase your weekly total. After you've adjusted to this volume of training, some faster paced training will help lower your times.

The first objective of faster paced training is not to improve your start or finish. Most runners seem to find a burst of speed at the beginning and end of races. The initial purpose of injecting faster paced running is to practice holding onto a faster pace in the middle 90% of a race. It doesn't have to be complicated. In fact, it can be a very simple change in the way you execute your Tuesday or Wednesday workout. Here's how it can work. After you have done your exercise routine and have fully warmed-up on your run, pick-up the pace for five minutes. As you start to tire, stay as smooth as you can until the five minutes are up. Slow the pace way down and recover at a slower pace for the next five minutes. Then surge again for another five minutes. Concentrate on maintaining the best stride and pace you can even if discomfort starts to set in. Slow down for five minutes. If you can manage, try to surge a third time. If you've already had enough, finish your run and cool down as you jog home. In a week or two, try to complete three surges. I know dozens of successful runners who have remained competitive for decades on this simple training formula. If you happen to run in a very demanding race, give yourself a few easy days to fully recover. Resume your normal training when you are ready. If you feel at home with the 10K distance but want to continue lowering your times, add another workout to your week by replacing a rest day with an easy running day. Beyond this level of training, you'll need to decide whether adding more speed or extra distance to your workouts will produce better results.

If you are a recreational runner with a goal to finish a half-marathon or full marathon, run farther for better results.

Follow the model of a more serious 10K runner and continue to gradually add one or two units of time/distance to your schedule. Increasing distance to your workouts will naturally take more time. It's important to make sure this extra time does not come at the expense of something important in your life. The life of a long distance runner is not for everyone. Before long, you will need to build up your daily/weekly totals by replacing rest days on your chart with additional days of easy running. Speed training is not a critical training element for recreational long distance runners just looking to finish a race. Once you've increased the distance of your long runs to 18k/11miles, or have adapted to training at a 50K/30miles per week level, you'll be ready to try a half-marathon. This will undoubtedly be less preparation than race winners have done. However, it should get you to the finish line. Running a half-marathon is a very respectable feat for any weekend racer. It is clearly an accomplishment requiring endurance, discipline, and fortitude. With that said, I understand the lure of what lies beyond. It might stem from the way 13.1 mile events are referred to as only "half".

Many have the impression your resume is incomplete, as a distance runner, until you've completed a "full" 26.2 mile marathon. You shouldn't feel that way. Marathoners are not the only true distance runners. However, if that's the way you feel, you should have a good idea what's in store before embarking on such a journey. In this author's opinion, you shouldn't attempt a full marathon until your body has adapted to training at a 100k/60miles per week level and your long runs have reached a minimum of 37k/23miles. If you truly enjoy training and altering your lifestyle to meet those prerequisites, you are indeed a marathoner at heart. It's possible to complete a marathon on less training, but you will most certainly experience a level of discomfort you won't soon forget.

Much has been written and said about what it takes to be successful at the marathon. Those in the know all agree that training needs to begin months in advance. It needs to be consistent and void of major injuries or illness. Training should taper the last few weeks before the race. Marathons should be followed by a period of rest and light training.

It doesn't take runners very long after a race to begin to wonder ... what's next?
After completing a marathon you'll know what it takes to run these longer distances well. Decide whether you enjoy training more for long distance endurance races or whether you prefer adding more speed to your runs. Perhaps your abilities and available training time are better suited for 5k to 10k races. You may also recognize that racing isn't your thing at all. You may discover that running alone, running with your dog, or running more casually with friends is all you need from the sport. Do what's right for you.

If your goal is to become a middle-distance track and field athlete, you will need to add more speed to your workouts. Physiologists say that an ideal miler/1500 meter runner should possess equal amounts of endurance and speed. Recognize that both components need to be developed and maintained. By the nature of what each component happens to represent, endurance takes longer to develop than speed. Endurance also takes more time to maintain throughout the year. Therefore, a miler/1500 meter runner should spend more time year-round running at a pace that will build endurance. Five thousand meter runners and steeplechasers, who jump thirty-five barriers while running three thousand meters, need two or three parts endurance for one part speed. That's why world class middle-distance runners spend a lot of time running at a steady pace, out on the roads and trails, similar to the way true long distance athletes train. This is called *aerobic* training, and occurs when breathing levels deliver enough oxygen to keep up with the muscles' demand.

As serious middle-distance runners get closer to their track racing season, they will begin to replace their longer runs with two or three days per week devoted to speed. The surges and recovery periods, known as intervals, will vary in duration and speed. The distance run and the time allowed to recover from each surge will vary depending on the goal of that workout. Runners trying to improve their raw speed will sprint for short distances and rest to nearly a full recovery before repeating. Those trying to develop sustained speed or stamina don't surge quite as fast but will start another surge before fully catching their breath. Both speed and stamina building workouts are examples of *anaerobic* training. This type of training occurs when the athlete's muscles are burning oxygen faster than the lungs and heart can keep up with the muscle's demand to deliver more oxygen. Athletes consuming oxygen at this rate go into *oxygen debt*. They are forced to activate an alternative energy system to compensate for this oxygen shortage. Although this alternative system is limited, it can be developed and extended with training. Middle-distance runners must learn to relax as much as possible as they fight through the burning buildup of lactic-acid created by this system. Athletes in oxygen debt experience a weird light-headed feeling that my friend, Ben Andrews, calls "lactic-acid wonderland". It soon goes away after the athlete catches his or her breath. High intensity speed workouts consume a lot of energy but in a different way compared to steady long distance runs. When either style is taken to extreme, adequate recovery needs to take place. The recovery from speed workouts and long runs is also a different process. Middle-distance runners shouldn't try to mix super long runs with super hard speed workouts in the same training phase. Super long runs should be done during the endurance phase of training. This phase should take place between a middle-distance racer's cross country and track seasons. As the speed work phase starts taking the place of longer runs, there should be a planned drop in longer runs and the overall distance run each week.

Coaches and self-coached individuals should design workout schedules to match the ability level, fitness level, and goals of each training group or athlete. Speed workouts are often timed on accurately measured tracks. Athletes will try to develop a sense of familiarity with the feel of the track and the running pace they will encounter in upcoming races. However, many famous champions have preferred working out on sandy beaches, grass parks, country roads, or trails. The difference being they surge for allotted time periods or from a given landmark to another. From a cardio-vascular standpoint, it doesn't really matter whether the training is done on or off a measured track. The main objective is to prepare the athlete for the rigors of racing while working to improve a specific aspect of the athlete's fitness or technique.

Successful middle-distance runners have been known to run multiple surges of the same distance in one session, for example; ten times four hundred meters with a one to three minute rest/recovery in-between surges. Sometimes they may vary the distances or length of time they surge, for example; surge for one hundred meters, jog one hundred, surge for two hundred meters, jog two hundred, surge for three hundred meters, jog three hundred, surge for four hundred meters, jog four hundred. This is known as a *ladder workout*. Once a runner has gone up the ladder they can come back down by repeating the surges and jogs in reverse order.

I've done regular repeating surge workouts as well as ladder workouts both on and off the track. Sometimes I time myself and sometimes I don't. Here's one of my favorite ways and places to do a workout when a track isn't available or nearby. I'll find a beautiful country road, without much traffic, and will use the telephone poles, fence posts, or mailboxes to signify the start of my surges and recovery jogs. I can run these sections in a predetermined order or mix it up as I go. My heart and lungs don't know the difference if the effort is the same. Just like finding the right stride, each athlete needs to discover the mixture and method of training that delivers the best individual results. **The true success of any type of training, which includes when, where, and how it took place, is measured in how well each athlete or team performs in competition.**

We've talked about improving your technique and having purpose in how you move. Understanding the relationship between exercise and recovery will also help you manage yourself to better performances and a better overall running experience. Training takes energy. Even if it makes you feel better afterward, energy has been spent and needs to be replaced. You have to eat, drink, and sleep to replenish the lost energy. One purpose of training is to get your body to adapt better to this cycle. As you adapt to this cycle, you'll be able to run faster and farther. Whether the goal is improved basic fitness or training for competition, most folks who run agree it is fun to be able to go faster and farther. Running with a fundamentally sound stride will help you do both.

As you practice and train, your strengths and your weaknesses will be revealed. This will show you that there is room for improvement. Knowing your areas for improvement should be encouraging, making you want to run more—with the added value of helping you develop your cardiovascular system. Motivation, satisfaction, fitness, health, and improved performance are all byproducts of working to improve your stride.

There's more to life than running for most of us and only so many hours in a day. That is why I believe in practicing the right way, being very specific about what you are trying to accomplish in every workout and ending a workout when you've had enough. These are all things I've learned the hard way. Hopefully, you will have a better understanding and pay better attention to the warning signs than I did. If you have big goals, you will have to work hard and be brave enough to really push your limits at times. But you will also have to be patient and smart enough to allow enough time for recovery, allowing your body to incorporate the training and to maintain your general health.

If you find yourself in poor shape as a result of an injury or layoff, you'll know right away. Remember, you didn't get out of shape in one day, so don't expect to become fit in only a day or two. Start off gradually and after a week or two, if it seems too easy, you can push yourself by adding some difficulty.

Balance Push with Rest in Your Schedule

Regardless of whether you are a beginner or a world-class athlete;

- Plan to run only two or three days a week farther *or* faster than normal.
- Allow two or three days a week to either rest completely or run less *and* easier than normal.

If some muscles get stiff or sore before others, something in your stride may be out of balance. This is a sign of overdoing one move and not doing enough of another. Over time, the result is a tightening of one group of muscles and often a weakening of others. When this happens, be proactive. Look for the problem in your stride or off-running activities, either on your own or with the help of someone with some expertise, before you end up in physical therapy. Running, walking, standing, or sitting too long can compress your body. Often the solution can be some alternative activity that counterbalances the effects of gravity. Many runners have great success with internal martial arts, like tai chi or yoga, because these activities involve stretching, better posture, improved balance, developing inner strength, and proper breathing. The key is to stretch and relax what is tight; strengthen what is weak; and understand your own body.

You need to work on things in a relaxed setting until they become second nature to your body and mind. This is best accomplished while under control at a slower speed. Gradually increase the speed as long as you can keep it fundamentally sound. Training partners need to understand when they should race or push each other and when to take it easy.

Knowing the What, How, and Why of Training

Assuming you are working toward a goal, you need to fully understand the process of your training. That means knowing what the workout of the day entails as well as knowing how and why you are doing it that way. For example, running nonstop for one hour would be *what* to do. Running at a steady pace, concentrating on good form, would be *how* to do it. Running steady for an hour fits into any runner's plan of increasing or maintaining endurance. This alone meets the reason *why*. Running at a steady, controlled pace is also a good time to work on needed changes in your form, giving you a bonus reason to *why* you are doing it.

Putting It All Together: A Note to Coaches

Here's one for you coaches out there with a team. Anyone can look up a bunch of workouts and fill them in on the calendar. In fact, let's say that cross-country coaches in the same league with similar kids are using the same workout schedule from the same book. Coach A has his kids running during the summer, and then starts the season with a team that is already in pretty good shape. Coach B is the kind that waits until the first day of school to see who's going to turn out. Coach C hates to lose at anything and believes that champions should always outwork their opponents. Coach C has the team running most of each workout as hard as they can and doesn't worry about form, because everyone knows how to run ... right?

The season progresses and Coach A has the team working out with an understanding of the *what*, *how*, and *why* they are doing things. Even if Coach B brings his team along—up to speed and using the same principles—they've simply lost too much ground from the beginning and won't be able to match the fitness and performance level of team A. How will Team C measure up?

Now, it's late in the season, a few days before the league championships. The scheduled workout for all three teams calls for ten repetitions of running 300 meters, with a 100-meter walk/jog after each one. Team C is tired, nursing injuries, and half of them are on the verge of catching a cold. They've worked so hard. In many ways, they deserve the trophy, but they are filled with anxiety. Deep down, most of them can't wait for the season to end. Their coach pushes them all to the brink of exhaustion, and he still hasn't announced who's running in the meet. The effort zaps their energy reserves and leaves them tired and/or sick by the day of the meet.

Team B has made steady progress throughout the season. They run the same workout hard, but save a little bit for the race on Thursday. As a group, they are gaining confidence and looking forward to the chance of finishing in the top two teams and earning a trip to the state meet.

By now, Team A is at their top fitness and running smooth. Coach A has them divide into groups according to ability. They take turns leading their packs, so they each know what it feels like to lead or follow at their own pace. No matter how the race unfolds, they will feel prepared and ready. On the last few repeats, they take turns being the leader for 200 meters and practice changing gears the last 100—to simulate sprinting and passing someone or holding their position on the homestretch. They are still working hard, but it's under control, working on several skills in one workout, each runner with an individual purpose, and an overall purpose for the team. This coach looks at each runner's progress and takes the time during breaks to teach individuals needing help. This is the way winning programs are built and reloaded with new talent year after year. Success only breeds success when it's done the right way.

Sure enough, Team A prevailed and they won another league championship. Up and down the roster, Team B matched up with their counterparts on Team C. With the right amount or positive energy and fresher legs, Team B surged man for man past the overtrained and worn-out members of Team C. The enthusiasm of Team B didn't vanish after earning their coveted trip to the state championship meet. The bulk of the team, sophomores and juniors, continued to train sensibly throughout the following year with goals of finishing higher. Their dedication and improvement allowed them to capture the league championship the next season and place higher at state.

A Final Thought from a Veteran of the Sport

For the most part, running is an individual activity. Even if you have running partners, teammates, or a coach, you are the one in charge of making each stride happen ... *and* choosing the form you want to use. When you start to get better, you will have breakthroughs. You will notice how a slight lean/tilt forward or upright, or the exact time you start a move, or the way your hips and knees are hinging in their sockets can affect your results. More important, you have learned *how it feels* when those things are occurring and how to make the necessary corrections.

Running has led me through good times and bad. After all these years, it's still fun to run fast and occasionally hear those cheers. I hope you hear many cheers as you *unleash your stride*.

> **For information about individual coaching and group clinics visit www.unleashyourstride.com.**